Writing Basics for the Healthcare Professional

Michele Benjamin Lesmeister, MA

Faculty, Basic Studies Department
Renton Technical College
Renton, Washington

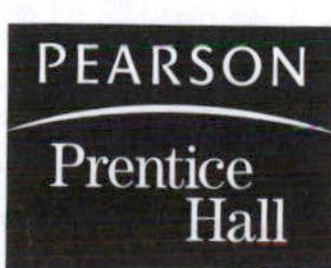

Upper Saddle River, New Jersey

Publisher: Julie Levin Alexander
Publisher's Assistant: Regina Bruno
Executive Editor: Mark Cohen
Associate Editor: Melissa Kerian
Managing Production Editor: Patrick Walsh
Production Management/Composition: Stratford Publishing Services
Production Editor: Margaret Pinette
Interior Design: Stratford Publishing Services
Director of Production and Manufacturing: Bruce Johnson
Manufacturing Manager: Ilene Sanford
Manufacturing Buyer: Pat Brown
Senior Design Coordinator: Christopher Weigand
Director of Marketing: Karen Allman
Marketing Manager: Harper Coles
Marketing Assistant: Wayne Celia
Marketing Coordinator: Michael Sirinides
Printer/Binder: Bind-Rite Graphics
Cover Design: Amy Rosen
Cover Photograph: © Brand X Pictures/Getty Images, Inc.
Cover Printer: Coral Graphics

Pearson Education LTD.
Pearson Education Australia PTY, Limited
Pearson Education Singapore, Pte. Ltd
Pearson Education North Asia Ltd
Pearson Education Canada, Ltd.
Pearson Educación de Mexico, S.A. de C.V.
Pearson Education—Japan
Pearson Education Malaysia, Pte. Ltd

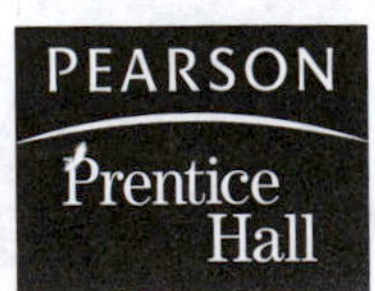

10 9 8 7 6 5 4 3 2 1
ISBN 0-8359-5319-X

For Albert, who believes in my work,
supports my intellectual endeavors,
and encourages my writing instruction.

Contents

Preface to Learners

Writing Basics for the Healthcare Professional is based on the writing needs of students in allied health fields. Over the past 15 years, many students in the allied health fields have asked me how to write for their programs. This book is designed to accomplish several objectives:

- build confidence through practice
- provide exams of real-life writing in the content field
- encourage professional communications
- model using medical terminology
- focus the basics of grammar in medical content

A wide variety of students will benefit from the "can-do" approach of this worktext. The answers for most of the exercises are at the end of the text. Proofreading and revision exercises help develop critical thinking skills in writing and a keen eye for written work. The self-checks are a measure of mastery.

Whether English is your first language or your second or third language, this worktext teaches the basic writing skills necessary to communicate effectively in the healthcare field. Practice is critical to your writing development, so the focus is on sentence structure. The medical terms at the beginning of each chapter provide a glance at the terms used in the unit exercises.

An instructor's guide complements the text and is available upon adoption. This guide provides a wealth of resources that will help facilitate instructional success. Features include:

- Unit notes with rationales for why the skill is being taught and its application in healthcare
- Teaching tips to encourage the reluctant or struggling writer
- Additional exercises that support the text and provide more sentence writing practice
- Additional unit extensions to offer learning options for extending the student's learning and application of writing skills
- Examinations designed to target the main skills of each chapter and promote practical writing skills
- Keys following each exam for scoring ease
- Reproducible rubrics matching those in the text ensure similar scoring guidelines

Reviewers

Norman Douglas Bradley
Lecturer, Writing Program
University of California
Santa Barbara, California

Nancy Dinsmore, COTA/L
Health Services Instructor
Green River Community College
Auburn, Washington

Janice C. Hess, MS
Director, Health Information Management Systems
Metropolitan Community College
Omaha, Nebraska

Jason C. Lira, MA
Instructor, English
Medical Careers Institute
Richmond, Virginia

Bradley Moore, MSN
Director, Health Science
Remington College
Little Rock, Arkansas

Ruth Ann O'Brien
Director of Allied Health
Miami Jacobs Career College
Dayton, Ohio

Kimberly M. Pearson, MS, RN
Adjunct Faculty
Illinois Central College
East Peoria, Illinois

Mary M. Prorok, RN, MSN
Instructor, Medical Office Specialist Program
South Hills School of Business and Technology
Altoona, Pennsylvania

Peg Rooney, RN, PhD
Regional Director
Colorado Community College and OccupationalEducation System
Denver, Colorado

Stewart R. Stanfield, MA
Professor, General Education
Platt College
Oklahoma City, Oklahoma

Acknowledgments

Special thanks to the contributers to this worktext:

Jade Benjamin-Chung, University of California, Berkeley, student in public health
Robert Do, University of Pennsylvania, business student
Jackie Elms, Licensed Practical Nurse
Tina Horner, Licensed Practical Nurse
Azeb Zeleke, Licensed Practical Nurse

UNIT 1

Grammar Basics

UNIT TERMS

Adjective	A word that describes a noun or a pronoun
Adverb	A word that describes a verb, adjective, or another adverb
Clause	A group of words that includes a subject and a verb; may be a dependent clause or an independent clause
Conjunction	A word or group of words that connects words or sentence parts
Describing word(s)	A word or group of words that describes or modifies other words
Grammar	The study of the structure or rules of language
Interjection	A word or group of words that expresses strong emotion
Modify	Describe or provide more information about something
Noun	A person place, thing, or idea
Phrase	A group of words that lacks a subject or a verb or both
Preposition	A word or group of words that shows a relationship between words
Pronoun	Any word that can take the place of a noun
Verb	A physical or mental action or a state of being

UNIT OBJECTIVES

Upon completion of this unit, the student should be able to

1. list the eight parts of speech
2. give the definition of grammar
3. define the eight parts of speech
4. edit to ensure correct use of the parts of speech
5. explain how grammar can benefit a writer

Glossary of Medical Terms

Term	Part of Speech	Definition
acne	noun	a disease of the oil glands that produces pimples and blackheads
apex	noun	the pointed end of a conelike structure
appendix	noun	an appendage of the digestive system
atherosclerosis	noun	the thickening and hardening of the arterial wall by cholesterol and triglyceride deposits

bacterium	noun	a one-celled organism without a nucleus
cancer	noun	a general term for malignant neoplasms or growths
carcinoma	noun	a malignant tumor
cardiac	adjective	pertaining to the heart
cardiologist	noun	a doctor specializing in heart disease
cauterize	verb	to burn with a cautery
diagnose; diagnosis	verb; noun	a method used to determine the cause and nature of a person's illness
endoscopy	noun	an internal inspection of body organs with an endoscope
excise	verb	to cut out or to remove by surgery
ganglion	noun	a mass of nervous tissue
gastric	adjective	relating to the stomach
incise	verb	to cut into
ingest	verb	to eat
lumen	noun	the space within an artery, intestine, or vein
lymphedema	noun	an abnormal swelling of tissue fluid
lymphoma	noun	a tumor in the lymph tissue
muscular	adjective	relating to muscles
neurologist	noun	a specialist in nervous system diseases
pediatrics	noun	the speciality of children's diseases and their treatment
pedometer	noun	a device for measuring infants; also an instrument that counts the number of steps taken
phlebotomist	noun	one who takes or draws blood
pleura	noun	a membrane that covers both lungs
radius	noun	the outer, shorter bone in the forearm
salivary	adjective	relating to the salivary glands
scrub	verb; noun	washing of the hands, nails, and upper arms before surgery
sedation	noun	a calm state; reduction of nervousness
spermatozoon	noun	a mature male sex cell
thorax	noun	the chest or area from base of neck to the diaphragm
urinalysis	noun	the analysis of urine
vertebra	noun	any of the 33 segments of the spinal column

EIGHT PARTS OF SPEECH

The eight parts of speech are the parts or components of grammar. The eight parts of speech work within the context of sentences. Each part of speech is used to determine the meaning and function of a specific word. Many English words can function as more than one part of speech. For example:

health (noun) Your health is important to your well-being.

In this example, *health* is functioning as a noun.

health (adjective) We will go to the health clinic to see the doctor.

Health is an adjective in this sentence. It is describing or modifying the noun *clinic*.

The parts of speech, as presented below, are ordered by relative importance to writing for health care.

NOUN

Definition: A noun is a person place, thing, activity, quality, or idea *(hospital, procedure, nurse, life, love, freedom, illness, oversight)*. Nouns can be common or proper. A common noun is a general noun and is not capitalized unless it begins a sentence. A proper noun is a specific name of something, and it is capitalized.

Common Nouns	Proper Nouns
doctor	Dr. Ito
tablet	Plavix
city	Los Angeles
faith	Catholic

Medical terms come from different languages. Many of the terms that we use today come from Latin and Greek. Latin and Greek provide the roots, suffixes, and the prefixes that we sometimes use to create new words. Medical terminology is based on these forms of language.

Knowing the suffixes that indicate nouns can be helpful in determining the form and function of a word. The suffix or final segment of most words in medical terminology determines the part of speech. This information is helpful for both writing sentences and proofreading. Knowing the definitions of suffixes allows one to spell the term correctly and choose the correct form of the medical term to use in each specific circumstance. Suffixes differentiate nouns from verbs and adjectives.

Suffix Indicating Noun	Definition of Suffix	Example	Definition
-ia	A condition or process	phobia	A condition of having fear
-ist	One who specializes in	urologist	One who specializes in urology
-ism, -y	A condition of or state of being	alcoholism; allergy	A condition of being an alcoholic; a condition of being allergic
-icle, -ole, -ula, -ule	Something little or small	venule, nodule	A small vein, a small node

Nouns usually show number by adding *–s* or *–es* for plurals, and they show possession by adding *'s* or *s'*. Some basic rules for forming plurals are presented in the chart below.

Rule for Forming Plurals	Examples
Add *–s* to most words in English to form plural form.	patient – patients doctor – doctors
When a singular word ends in *s, sh, ch, x,* or *z*, add *–es* to form the plural.	class – classes box – boxes
When a singular word ends in *ay, ey, oy,* or *uy*, add *–s* to form the plural.	key – keys alley – alleys

(continued)

Rule for Forming Plurals	Examples
When a singular word ends in a consonant +*y*, change the *y* to *i* and add –*es* to form the plural.	baby – babies cry – cries
Some words change their spelling and form; these must be memorized.	child – children man – men
For some words that end in *f*, change the *f* to *v* and add –*es* to form the plural. For other words that end in *f*, just add –*s* for plural forms.	thief – thieves leaf – leaves grief – griefs
For some hyphenated words, add –*s* to the main part of the word to form the plural.	mother-in-law – mothers-in-law
For words ending in *o*, either add –*s* or –*es* to form the plural.	potato – potatoes photo – photos

These singular-to-plural forms are learned over time and may be checked in a dictionary.

In health care, sometimes nouns are pluralized in different ways, such as by changing the suffix at the end of the root word. This is because the plurals are formed by the rules of Latin or Greek. Some examples are given below.

Singular	Singular Ending	Plural	Plural Ending	Rule for Forming the Plural
vertebra	*a*	vertebrae	*ae*	Keep the *a* and add *e*.
thorax	*x*	thoraces	*ces*	Remove the *x* and add *ces*.
lumen	*en*	lumina	*ina*	Remove *en* and add *ina*.
urinalysis	*is*	urinalyses	*es*	Remove *is* and add *es*.
appendix	*ex* or *ix*	appendices	*ices*	Remove *ex* or *ix* and add *ices*.
spermatozoon	*on*	spermatozoa	*a*	Remove *on* and add *a*.
bacterium	*um*	bacteria	*a*	Remove *um* and add *a*.
radius	*us*	radii	*i*	Remove *us* and add *i*.
cavity	*y*	cavities	*ies*	Remove *y* and add *ies*.
lymphoma	*ma*	lymphomata	*mata*	Keep the *ma* and add *ta*.

EXERCISE 1-1: Fill in the chart with the correct form to make these words singular or plural.

Singular	Plural
	carcinomata
ganglion	
apex	
	diagnoses
	pleurae

Nouns have specific functions. These functions are important for understanding sentence order and structure. These functions are provided below.

Functions	Examples
Subjects of sentences	*The nurse called the family. Insurance policies are often difficult to understand without careful reading.*
Objects of prepositions	*The duties of the volunteer were to locate and provide magazines to the patients.*
Appositive phrases	*The procedure, an upper digestive tract endoscopic examination, requires sedation.*
	The woman purchased a new device, a pedometer.
Predicate nominatives	*He became a licensed practical nurse.*
	The doctor is a cardiologist.
Direct objects	*The nurse gave Sally a form to complete.*
(receive the verb's action)	*Hospitals mail bills monthly.*
Indirect objects	*The nurse gave Sally a form to complete.*
(receive the direct object)	*The medical office mails patients their bills.*

EXERCISE 1-2: Read the passage below; then underline each noun.

Many herbs and vitamins have shown new hope for treating diabetes. There is some concern for the safety and efficacy of herbal remedies. It may be too soon for experts to make recommendations about most of these herbs and vitamins, but the medical community is showing some interest in these alternative approaches to healthcare.

EXERCISE 1-3: Write sentences with the following common nouns.

1. pediatrics

____

____

2. acne

____

____

3. tension

____

____

4. surgeon

____

____

5. cancer

____

____

EXERCISE 1-4: Underline the subject in the following sentences.

1. The amputation—a partial or complete removal of a limb—was performed by the medical team in the military hospital.
2. A fracture indicates a breakage of a bone by disease or trauma.
3. His condition of gout has caused acute arthritis and joint inflammation.
4. Your insulin, used to treat diabetes, will lower your glucose levels.
5. Her osteoplasty is scheduled for early June.

Other examples of nouns in health professions are the titles of medical specialists and their fields of practice. These are both nouns, but they are generally given in two forms:

Noun root word + *ist* is the specialist.

Noun root word + *ology* is the field of specialty.

By building a chart of specialist, field or practice, and type of care provided, writers can quickly learn the scope of each area of specialty and build a basis for additional learning.

Specialist	Field or Practice of Specialty	Type of Care Provided
dermatologist	dermatology	diagnoses and treats patients with skin disorders
gerontologist	gerontology	diagnoses and treats aging patients
neurologist	neurology	diagnoses and treats patients' nervous system disorders
oncologist	oncology	diagnoses and treats patients with tumors
pediatrician	pediatrics	diagnoses and treats diseases in children

EXERCISE 1-5: Complete the chart with specialists and fields.

Specialist	Field or Practice of Specialty	Type of Care Provided
	endocrinology	treatment of disease of the endocrine glands
anesthesiologist		administration of anesthesia to patients to create partial or complete loss of sensation
	pharmacology	dispensing of prescribed medications
	immunology	treatment of diseases of the immune system
endodontist		diagnoses, treatment, and prevention of diseases of the dental pulp and surrounding tissues
	otolaryngology	treatment of ear, nose, and throat diseases
orthodontist		prevention and correction of misaligned teeth

	ophthalmology	treatment of disorders of the eye
	gynecology	treatment of diseases specific to women
osteopath		treatment of diseases of the bone

PRONOUN

Definition: A pronoun is a word that can replace a noun. Pronouns may be subjects, objects, or words showing possession. Personal pronouns relate to a specific person *(he, she, them, us, we)*. Some pronouns refer to nouns in general; these are called indefinite pronouns *(anyone, each, somebody)*. Other pronouns point out particular objects *(that, this, these, those)*. There are also pronouns that introduce questions *(who, which, what)*.

Functions	Examples
As a subject	*<u>He</u> was screened as a bone marrow donor.*
As an object	*The lab mailed <u>her</u> the report.*
As a way to show possession	*That assignment is <u>hers</u>. The nurse gave <u>his</u> mother a hug.*

The chart below serves to provide the form and function of each pronoun.

Subject Pronouns	Object Pronouns	Possessive Pronouns	
• Subjects of sentence • Predicate nominatives	• Direct objects • Indirect objects • Objects of the preposition	• These pronouns are followed by a noun.	• These pronouns refer to a noun given in the sentence.
I	me	my	mine
he	him	his	his
she	her	her	hers
it	it	its	its
you	you	your	yours
we	us	our	ours
they	them	their	theirs
who	whom	whose	whose

Here are some examples:

The technician prepared the equipment; <u>he</u> is in charge of assisting others in the lab.

<u>Who</u> will meet with the family to discuss the patient care plan?

The nurse put <u>his</u> X-ray on the viewing screen.

The doctor is in responding to <u>her</u> patient.

Those insurance papers are <u>theirs</u>.

Exercise 1-6: Use these pronouns in sentences.

1. our

___

___

2. whose

___

___

3. they

___

___

4. yours

___

___

5. her

___

___

Certain indefinite pronouns may be singular or plural. The table below shows which indefinite pronouns are singular, plural, or can function as both singular and plural.

Singular	Plural	Singular or Plural
someone, somebody, something	both	all
anyone, anybody, anything	few	any
everyone, everybody, everything	many	half
no one, nobody, nothing	several	most
every		none
one		some
each		
another		

Exercise 1-7: Write sentences with these pronouns.

1. everything

___

___

2. each

___

___

3. few

4. most

5. half

VERB

Definition: A verb is a physical or mental action or process or a state of being, and it is part of the predicate. A predicate is the verb and its complements or verb-related words.

All verbs are either action verbs *(remove, incise, lift)* or linking verbs *(is, are, am, been, became, seem)*. A verb may be part of a verb phrase that has more than one verb and provides information on tense (the time of the action) and voice (active or passive) for the sentence. For example:

The nurse *prepares* the medication. (verb)

The patient *seems* agitated. (linking verb)

The medical team *will meet* with the family. (verb phrase)

Functions	Examples
Verbs	*The nurse relied on the family for patient information.* (action verb)
	The patient was irritated by the tests. (linking verb)
Verbals	*Preparing the examination rooms is his chief duty.*

Verbs acting as other parts of speech are covered in Unit 6: Achieving More in Sentence Variety.

Hint: Ask yourself, "The subject or the actor in the sentence did what?" to locate the verb. For example: The nurse poured the medication into the tablespoon. The nurse did what? The nurse *poured* the medication. So, *poured* is the action, and it is the verb of this sentence.

LINKING VERB OR ACTION VERB?

It is important to be able to differentiate a linking verb from an action verb. A linking verb may be followed by either an adjective, a prepositional phrase, or a noun. Common linking verbs include *am, is, are, was, were, seems, become, and appear*. Linking verbs are used to describe or rename the subject. For example:

Mary ***is*** *in the hospital waiting room.* (prepositional phrase)

The surgeon ***appeared*** *gentle and understanding.* (adjectives)

My neighbor ***is*** *a neurologist.* (noun)

Action verbs are used to indicate physical actions. They are modified by adverbs that complete the action by indicating when, where, how, or to what extent the action is done:

The dental assistant prepared the instruments carefully.
(verb) (adverb)

The hospital staff evacuated the patients efficiently.
(verb) (adverb)

This knowledge about verbs is critical when one must decide which form of a describing word to choose. Follow these steps:

1. Locate the verb.
2. Determine if it is a linking verb (state of being) or an action verb (physical or mental activity).
3. Decide if the modifying word should be an adverb or an adjective.

Action verbs are described with adverbs:

The mole grew (irregular, irregularly).

Locate the verb *grew*, which is the action of the subject *mole*, so *grew* is an action verb. Then, choose the adverb, *irregularly:*

The mole grew irregularly.

The patient's family is supportive of the care she is receiving.

Locate the verb *is*. This verb shows the state of being for the family. So *is* is a linking verb, and it requires an adjective, *supportive*.

EXERCISE 1-8: Identify the verb and underline the verb type for each sentence. Then underline the correct modifying word in parentheses for each sentence.

Verb Types	Examples
1. Action or Linking Verb	The disturbed resident yelled (loud, loudly).
2. Action or Linking Verb	The LPN student performed (good, well) at his clinical site.
3. Action or Linking Verb	The doctor could (sure, surely) order the tests.
4. Action or Linking Verb	The surgical team looked (tired, tiredly) after the 12 hours of work.
5. Action or Linking Verb	The family seems (unhappy, unhappily) with the diagnosis.
6. Action or Linking Verb	Today, the patient felt (good, well) after the examination and medical tests.

Exercise 1-9: Write sentences that incorporate these verbs. Refer to the unit glossary for definitions of these words.

1. excise

____

____

2. cauterize

____

____

3. diagnose

____

____

4. incise

____

____

5. instruct

____

____

ADJECTIVE

Adjectives are modifying or describing words. These words help readers understand nouns. Adjectives provide descriptions that include color, shape, size, form, number, kind, and so on of a noun.

Definition: An adjective is a word that describes a noun or pronoun *(sweet, healthful, irritated, enlarged, seven, friendly)*: That diet is healthful. Your dietary choices can influence your emotional state.

Functions	Examples
Modifies or describes a noun	*The tubal irrigation was performed by the nurse. The endoscopic procedure lasted about one hour.*
Modifies or describes a pronoun	*He was incoherent. His wound was invasive.*

Hint: Ask yourself, "What kind of _____? How many? What size?" to locate the adjectives. These questions help point to the modifying or descriptive words or adjectives.

Exercise 1-10: Read the passage below, then underline each adjective.

Recently, the medical community has discussed the need for all people to reduce the fat in their diets. The fast food industry has supersized portions that encourage people to overeat. Today many people are reducing the amount of food that they ingest. By reducing their intake, individuals hope to extend their healthy years.

In the medical field, certain suffixes generally indicate that the word is an adjective, as given below.

Suffix	Example	Definition
-ac	cardiac	pertaining to the heart
-al	dermal	pertaining to the skin
-ary	salivary	pertaining to the saliva glands
-ar	muscular	pertaining to a muscle
-ic	gastric	pertaining to the stomach

EXERCISE 1-11: Write a sentence with each adjective. Refer to unit glossary for definitions of these words.

1. cardiac

____

____

2. dermal

____

____

3. salivary

____

____

4. muscular

____

____

5. gastric

____

____

ADVERB

Definition: An adverb is a word that describes a verb, adjective, or other adverb by providing how, to what extent, or under what condition *(solemnly, uniformly, too, really, kindly).*

Functions	Examples
Describes a verb	*The scrub was performed quietly. (how?)*
Describes an adjective	*The medical records were very detailed. (to what extent?)*
Describes another adverb	*The trauma team was really very tired. (to what extent?)*

Hint: To locate the adverb, ask yourself, "Verb how? When was the action taken? Under what condition? Or to what extent was something done?"

The call came immediately after the patient reached the hospital.

When did the call come? *Immediately*. So *immediately* is the adverb.

The long-term care administrator was quite amicable with family and staff.

How amicable was the long-term care administrator? *Quite*. So *quite* is an adverb.

EXERCISE 1-12: Read the passage below, then underline each adverb.

Phoenix, Arizona, has a very big problem this year. According to health officials, the state is the only state where the mosquito-borne West Nile virus has already reached an epidemic. Arizona has a lot of standing water in the form of pools and irrigation ditches. This water effectively harbors these insects. So far, there have been 290 cases of West Nile virus in Arizona this year. State officials are very worried that as many as 300,000 Arizonans might have the virus; they may not know it yet. The officials are carefully monitoring the situation.

EXERCISE 1-13: Use the following adverbs in a sentence.

1. rather

____

____

2. here

____

____

3. not

____

____

4. then

____

____

5. cautiously

____

____

PREPOSITION

Definition: A preposition is a word or group of words that shows the relationship between words in a sentence *(with, of, among)*. A prepositional phrase consists of a preposition and its object, which is a noun or pronoun *(to surgery, for the nurse, in the dental lab)*.

Common prepositions include the following:

about	aside from	during	next	through
above	at	except	of	throughout
across	because	for	off	to
after	before	from	on	toward
against	behind	in	onto	under
along	below	inside	out	until
among	between	into	outside	up
around	by	like	over	with
as	down	near	since	without

Prepositions are primarily used in prepositional phrases, which are prepositions + nouns, or prepositions + pronouns.

Functions	Examples
Describes time:	*The procedure was done in under the two hours.*
Describes place:	*The mole removal was done in an outpatient clinic.*
Describes direction:	*Wipe the opening in a circular motion.*

Note: Prepositional phrases never function as the subjects in a sentence. In the examples below, the subjects are underlined and the prepositional phrases are in brackets [ ].

Some [of the children] still need their vaccinations.

Many [of the insurance forms] were outdated.

Each [of the staff members] participates in planning patient care.

Hint: Ask yourself, "Where? When?" to locate the prepositional phrases. For clear expression, place the prepositional phrase as close to the noun it modifies or describes.

EXERCISE 1-14: Read the passage below, then underline each prepositional phrase.

A certified nursing assistant (CNA) is an entry-level caregiver. The job duties of a CNA are varied. Much of the difficult tasks are completed by these dedicated and caring individuals. They are trained in personal hygiene, first aid, care giving, bed making, and feeding techniques. From morning to night, patients rely on their assistance. Sometimes, a senior citizen may have only a CNA who pays attention to his or her daily needs. Thus, the value of the role of the certified nursing assistant should not be taken for granted.

EXERCISE 1-15: Write sentences that include these prepositional phrases.

1. beside the examination table

____

____

2. for the laboratory procedure

____

____

3. in trauma cases

____

____

4. under the doctor's care

____

____

5. among the bandages

____

____

CONJUNCTION

Definition: A conjunction is a word or phrase that connects or joins individual words or groups of words, phrases, and clauses.

Function: There are three types of conjunctions: coordinating, correlative, and subordinating. There are seven coordinating conjunctions: *and, but, or, yet, so, for*, and *nor*. Coordinating conjunctions are words that join equal grammatical units. For example:

The patient felt depressed and dejected. (adjective and adjective)

The director of the long-term care center is hiring many staff members, for she needs to ensure adequate staffing to meet state requirements. (sentence and sentence)

Subordinating conjunctions are words that join two clauses that are not equal in importance. In other words, a subordinating conjunction is used to join an independent and a dependent clause. Some examples of subordinating conjunctions are *after, although, as, as long as, because, so that, since, until, when, where*, and *while*.

> Although the patient tried to walk, he was unable to bear his weight for long.
>
> The physical therapist worked hard to help the stroke victim because he realized that the patient's independence was at stake.

EXERCISE 1-16: Read each sentence. Underline the conjunction and write the type of conjunction on the blank line. Use these labels: coordinating conjunction (cc), correlative conjunction (corr), or subordinating conjunction (sc).

1. Because depression is prominent on college campuses, college counselors are using more interventions to assist students. ________
2. The students wanted to research the disease, so the professor gained access to the data for them. ________
3. The more she worked on her medical terminology, the more proficient she became as a medical receptionist. ________
4. Lyme disease can make some people feel fatigued and in pain, while others suffer depression, anxiety, and memory loss. ________
5. The disease started with a rash, and it was followed with flulike symptoms. ________

EXERCISE 1-17: Use each of the conjunctions in a sentence.

1. while

____

____

2. as if

____

____

3. but

____

____

4. before

____

____

5. not only . . . but also

____

____

INTERJECTION

Definition: Interjections are words and phrases that are used to show strong expression or emotion. Punctuation is used to separate the expression from another sentence. Some examples of interjections are *oh well, yes, absolutely*, and *hey*.

Function: Interjections would not normally be used in writing as a healthcare professional, with one exception: A writer might include an interjection when documenting a patient's communication or when providing an example of how the patient communicated information.

Hey! I need you to turn the light on.

Oh no! I have the wrong medical chart.

Parts of speech can help writers associate words in families. The chart below shows the writer the correct form of the word for the intended purpose. Notice that not all words have all three word forms; in this case, an *X* is used to indicate that no form exists.

For example:

The nurse insisted on Mr. Wallace's ambulation. (noun)

He will ambulate the length of the hallway. (verb)

His ambulatory stance creates a balance problem, which is a safety issue. (adjective)

Noun	Verb	Adjective
ambulation	ambulate	ambulatory
endoscopy	*X*	endoscopic
diagnosis	diagnose	diagnostic
internist	intern	internal
alcohol, alcoholism	*X*	alcoholic
thorax	*X*	thoracic
hemorrhage	hemorrhage	hemorrhaging
atrophy	atrophy	atrophic, atrophied
aphasia	*X*	aphasic

EXERCISE 1-18: Add an ending or suffix to each word to make the desired form of the word. Endings to be used to complete the table are *-ment, -ed, -ate, -ion,*

and *-tic*. Fill in the correct form of the word. If none exists, use an *X* in the box to indicate that none exists. Some words may change spelling.

Noun	Verb	Adjective
	depress	
vaccination		
		medicated
	incise	
		enriched
spasm		

PHRASES

A phrase is a group of words that work together for a purpose, but a phrase lacks a subject, a verb, or both a subject and a verb. Phrases usually modify other words in some way.

In English we have several kinds of phrases that can help us communicate our ideas. Prepositional phrases and verb phrases will be covered in this unit. Appositive, gerund, infinitive, and participial phrases are covered in Unit 6, Achieving More in Sentence Variety.

A **prepositional phrase** is a group of words that begins with a preposition and ends in a noun or pronoun. Prepositional phrases usually function as adjectives or adverbs; for example, *in the clinic, for the patient, with the medical assistant.*

EXERCISE 1-19: Complete the following prepositional phrases.

1. of ______________________________
2. against ___________________________
3. except ____________________________
4. after _____________________________
5. between ___________________________

A **verb phrase** is a group of verbs that consists of helping verbs (auxiliary verbs) and a main verb. Verb phrases provide the time and meaning of the action or state given by the main verb. The final verb in the phrase is the main verb or action verb, and all the preceding verbs are the helping verbs; these helping verbs form the time and meaning for the verb's action or state; for example, *will be incised, has sutured, is interviewing, had broken.*

EXERCISE 1-20: Underline each verb and verb phrase.

The hospital assistant is making Mr. Anderson's bed and preparing for his return. The patient is completing some X-rays on the first floor. Then he will return for a brief rest. Thereafter, he will complete a session of occupational therapy on the fifth floor. Rehabilitation requires daily exercise and adherence to a specific plan. Mr. Anderson is usually motivated to complete his exercises each day. He is tired at the end of each session with the physical therapist. He is progressing well with his treatment plan and will be released before the weekend.

EXERCISE 1-21: Use each of the verb phrases in a complete sentence.

1. will repeat

____

____

2. has diagnosed

____

____

3. has lost

____

____

4. will be removed

____

____

5. have felt

____

____

CLAUSES

A clause is a group of words that includes a subject and a verb. There are two types of clauses, independent (main) and dependent (subordinate) A clause is independent if it can stand alone as a sentence. Dependent clauses generally begin with subordinating conjunctions such as *although, if, since,* and *when.* A dependent clause can never stand alone as a sentence; it must be attached to an independent clause to form a complete sentence. For example:

The nurse was assigned to the west wing of the hospital. (independent)

Because the nurse was delivering a chart (dependent)

<u>Since the patient was given the medication</u>, she was able to tolerate the pain. (dependent clause + independent clause)

The long-term care facility worked hard to accommodate both single and married residents, <u>although this required a larger facility and separate living quarters</u>. (independent clause + dependent clause)

More work with clauses will be accomplished in Unit 3, which drafts different sentence types based on clause combinations.

Exercise 1-22: Finish the clauses to create an independent clause or sentence.

1. The patient ______________________________
2. The tissue ______________________________
3. The phlebotomist ______________________________
4. Seeing the therapist ______________________________
5. After the consultation, ______________________________

Exercise 1-23: Write a sentence that includes these subordinating conjunctions.

1. Because ______________________________
____
2. Since ______________________________
____
3. Until ______________________________
____
4. ______________________________ whenever ______
____
5. ______________________________ before
____

UNIT PROOFREADING EXERCISES

Read the passage below and make the corrections by crossing out the errors; then replace each error with the correction.

Ms. Robinswood wants to visit her doctor. Three year ago she had three sarcoma removed. She believes everyone should see their doctor once a year. One of her friends agrees with she; however, most don'. They believe they are healthy. Ms. Robinswood is caution about her health. Because she had cancer one times before, she is more careful than her friends. She appears health, but she just wants to make sure she is well.

UNIT REVISION EXERCISES

Read the sentences below and correct the form of the underlined word so that the correct form of the medical terminology is used in each sentence.

1. The gauze formed a <u>protect</u> layer.
2. The <u>psychology</u> will now see the patient.

3. She will excision the tumor.
4. Ambulation the patient this morning.
5. The surgery was invade.
6. The oncology will see new patients; she has expanded her practice.
7. Five patients had urinalysis completed by the laboratory technician this morning.
8. Doctors' diagnosis sometimes vary, based on experience and training.

Revise this sentence to make it a complete sentence.

9. Because he is worried about recurrence.

____

____

Correct the grammatical error in the following sentence.

10. The consultation with Dr. Ishmel is important for you and I.

____

____

UNIT EXTENSIONS

1. Review a medical journal or health-related magazine article from an online source or website. Print it. Then underline all the medical terminology. Label these words with their parts of speech.
2. Go to a website that has medical information, such as www.webmd.com. Find an article of interest. Review the language in the article. Print the article and underline all the prepositional phrases and the prepositional phrases.
3. Describe your state of well-being. Use all the parts of speech. Underline all the dependent clauses and then label each noun and verb.

UNIT 1 SELF-CHECK

Label each underlined word with its part of speech. Use adjective, adverb, conjunction, interjection, noun, pronoun, preposition, and verb.

_______________ 1. Atherosclerosis, a form of arteriosclerosis, is a degenerative vascular disorder.

_______________ 2. The specialist will call the patient as soon as the blood work is reviewed.

_______________ 3. Lyme disease can be an undetected illness.

_______________ 4. Mice suddenly lost weight when injected with leptin.

_______________ 5. Inflammation is a main mechanism in heart disease.

______________ **6.** Because so many factors were involved in his treatment, a team of medical staff worked together to form a plan.

Underline the phrases in the sentence below.

7. Now the medical community has gained more knowledge about the complexity of this disease as a result of the research provided by the Centers for Disease Control.

Underline the main clause in each sentence below.

8. The condition of the patient is improving, which has made the family hopeful.

9. Because the drug is still in the experimental stage, it is unavailable to the general public.

10. Insects that carry parasites often infect people through vector sites.

UNIT 2

Sentence Basics

UNIT TERMS

Article	*A, an, the;* used as adjectives
Clause	A group of words that includes a subject and a verb; may be dependent clause or independent clause
Command	A sentence that makes a request for action; also called an imperative
Exclamatory sentence	A sentence that show strong emotion, feeling, or need for action
Imperative sentence	A sentence that makes a request for action; also called a command
Interrogative sentence	A sentence that asks a question; also called a question
Predicate	The action or state of being of the subject; also called the verb
Question	A sentence that asks a question; also called an interrogative sentence
Subject	Who or what the sentence is about; the person, thing, or concept that is doing the verb's action
Sentence	A group of words that includes a subject and predicate and expresses a complete thought
Sentence fragment	An incomplete thought that is missing at least one essential part of a sentence

UNIT OBJECTIVES

Upon completion of this unit, the student should be able to

1. list the essential parts of a sentence
2. correctly punctuate a sentence
3. identify a sentence fragment
4. punctuate simple sentences
5. identify the four types of sentences

Glossary of Medical Terms

Term	Part of Speech	Definition
aseptic	adjective	sterile, clean, without germs
autopsy	noun	an after-death examination of tissue and organs to determine the cause of death
bifurcate	verb; adjective	divide into two parts or to split

calibrate	verb	to adjust a measurement or equipment for accuracy
elicit	verb	call forth, bring out, or evoke
grievance	noun	a complaint or resentment
incubate	verb	to keep in a controlled environment to keep something alive
intubate	verb	to insert a tube into a place like the throat
ligate	verb	to tie or bind
myalgia	noun	muscle pain or tenderness
palpate	verb	to examine by touch or feel
prenatal	adjective	before birth
salmonella	noun	a bacterial infection caused by eating raw or contaminated food; affects the gastrointestinal tract
suture	verb; noun	to sew together; also, the line of union of skull bones or other bones

DEFINITION OF A SIMPLE SENTENCE

A sentence is a group of words that communicates a complete idea. There are essential parts to every sentence: subject, predicate (verb), expression of a complete thought. One set of these essential parts of a sentence creates one main clause or one simple sentence. Sentences have other rules, too. The first word in a sentence is capitalized, and the sentence ends is some form of punctuation. Sentences are the basic units from which paragraphs and essays are built.

PARTS OF A SIMPLE SENTENCE

Sentences express a complete thought, begin with a capital letter, and end with a mark of punctuation. Sentences have the following parts: a subject, which is stated or implied, and a predicate.

1. *Subject (stated or implied):* Subjects are who or what is completing the verb's actions. A subject may be stated or implied (not obvious or given). When a subject is stated, it is given in the sentence. For example:

   This patient needs a referral to a neurologist.

   The nurses and medical assistants are meeting to discuss a plan of care.

   The subject is often the first noun in the sentence; however, this is not always the case. Sometimes an adverb such as *here* or *there* or a prepositional phrase comes first in the sentence. Then the subject will often be after the predicate:

   There is a pharmaceutical sales representative waiting to see the doctor.

   Here waits your patient.

   Implied subjects most often occur in the form of commands. This does not mean that the group of words is a fragment. Instead, a writer will recognize that the sentence starts with a verb and does not end in a question mark; thus, it is usually a command or request for someone to do something. For example:

Open the cabinet slowly. [*You* is the implied subject.]

Remove the sutures tomorrow. [*You* is the implied subject.]

2. *Predicate (verb):* The predicate provides the action or state of being for the subject. The verb is part of the predicate. The predicate provides the time the verb takes place (tense):

   The patient seems preoccupied. (present time)

   We will meet with the psychiatrist. (future time)

3. *Expression of a complete thought:* A sentence must express a complete thought:

   Because you need stitches. (incomplete thought)

   We will go to the emergency room because you need stitches. (complete thought)

   When a sentence does not express a complete thought, this is a serious error. It may confuse the reader.

4. *Capitalization of the first word:* All simple sentences begin with a capital letter:

   The medical assistant took the patient's blood pressure.

   Can you hold still as I take this X-ray?

   Call the next of kin.

5. *End punctuation:* A sentence ends with a punctuation sign. The sign depends on the type of sentence. Punctuation for sentences includes a period (.), a question mark (?), or an exclamation point (!). Sentence types are discussed a little later in the unit:

   I will remove the staples. (sentence)

   Do you feel pain? (question)

   Suction the patient in Room 212! (Exclamation)

   Remove the bandage, please. (Command)

If a sentence does not include these five items (subject, verb, complete thought, capitalized first word, and end punctuation), the sentence will have errors in grammar or mechanics.

SENTENCE FRAGMENTS

A writer may create a sentence fragment, which is only part of a sentence. This type of error is considered serious because it creates confusion. Most commonly, a sentence fragment is created when one of these essential sentence parts is missing: subject, verb, or expression of a complete thought. A simple sentence can include a subject and a verb but still be a sentence fragment if it begins with a subordinating conjunction.

EXERCISE 2-1: Indicate if the sentence is a complete sentence (CS) or a fragment (F)

1. ______ The doctor seems.
2. ______ The workplace is stressful, so we need to have hobbies to relax.
3. ______ Because of the way that the man and woman argued in front of the nurses.
4. ______ The diagnosis was made after many tests.
5. ______ Consulting with one another was the medical team.
6. ______ By caring for your eyesight, you will retain your excellent vision.
7. ______ For me, I need reassurance that I will be healthy again.
8. ______ The drugs are powerful.
9. ______ Avoid the dangerous streets; stay home tonight.
10. ______ The patient with his leg in a cast.

EXERCISE 2-2: Underline the subject once and the verb twice.

1. Our relationship with food changes over time.
2. Many people now avoid trans fats in their diets.
3. Remember to relax.
4. Carbohydrates provide most of our calories.
5. In the average American diet, carbohydrates make up about 50% of our calories.
6. The secret to making good coffee is in the bean.
7. The doctor and nurses are in a staff meeting.
8. The patient must sign the medical release form.
9. Her condition is becoming progressively worse.
10. Your insurance card will be mailed to your home address.

COMPOUND SUBJECTS AND PREDICATES

The simple sentence consists of one main clause. This main clause may have modifying words or groups of words, but it will have no other clauses. Examples of simple sentences are:

The nurse appeared confident.

The blood test was negative.

By early afternoon, the patient felt better.

Ketoacidosis, a diabetic coma, may develop over several days.

Sometimes a sentence includes more than one subject and more than one verb. Compound subjects and/or compound verbs are not separate clauses, but rather they expand the scope of the subject, verb, or both. As long as the two subjects or verbs are the ones doing the specific action in the simple sentence, a compound subject or verb has not changed the classification of sentence. Below are examples of sentences with compound subjects and verbs:

The patient and her family were elated at the test results. (compound subject)

Neuroglia contain and support nervous tissue. (compound verb)

The doctors and nurses planned and implemented the patient care plans. (compound subject and compound verb)

EXERCISE 2-3: Write a simple sentence of your own with each of the following terms. Refer to unit glossary for definitions of these words.

1. prenatal

___

___

2. salmonella

___

___

3. grievance

___

___

4. myalgia

___

___

5. managed care

___

___

EXERCISE 2-4: Use these compound subjects and verbs in sentences of your own.

1. purchase and restock

___

___

2. Dr. Smith and Dr. Halle

____

____

3. prescribed and filled

____

____

4. clean and suture

____

____

5. compare and sort

____

____

FOUR TYPES OF SENTENCES

A sentence comes in four forms: simple sentence, command, question, and exclamation.

SIMPLE SENTENCE

A simple sentence or declarative sentence is a sentence that consists of one main clause. Each main clause includes a subject and a verb, expresses a complete thought, and has initial capitalization and end punctuation.

A hernia is a protrusion of an organ through its cavity wall.

People experience different degrees of heartburn.

COMMAND OR IMPERATIVE SENTENCE

A command or imperative sentence gives a command or makes a request. The subject is generally understood; this type of sentence most often begins with a verb.

Fax this prescription to (360) 555-0100.

Consider seeing a dietitian right away.

A command is used in informal writing and oral communication. This type of sentence is not often seen in formal professional writing.

QUESTION OR INTERROGATIVE SENTENCE

An interrogative sentence asks a question. This type of sentence ends in a question mark. It also usually begins with a verb or a questioning word like *how, what, which*, or *who*.

How can I research this medication?

What does ADA stand for?

Is Dr. Tuttle on call this weekend?

EXCLAMATORY SENTENCE

An exclamatory sentence communicates strong emotion or urgent feelings. Most often these sentences will end in an exclamation point (!).

Prepare for surgery now!

Those flowers are gorgeous!

Give 5 grains of morphine STAT!

Call 911!

This patient is looking great!

Rarely will these sentence types occur in formal professional writing.

EXERCISE 2-5: State whether each of the following sentences is a simple sentence (SS), a command (Com), a question (Qu), or an exclamatory sentence (Ex). Write the answer on the line provided.

______ **1.** Contact the hospice coordinator at (425) 555-0100.

______ **2.** Is there an operating room available now?

______ **3.** Sign your legal name on this insurance form.

______ **4.** Esophagitis can be treated easily.

______ **5.** Will this medication decrease my appetite?

______ **6.** Call the head nurse STAT!

______ **7.** What a lovely day!

______ **8.** Your daughter is recovering quickly.

______ **9.** When will the doctor sign the release papers?

______ **10.** Please remove your glasses.

EXERCISE 2-6: Write one sentence of your own in each type below.

1. simple sentence

____

____

2. command

____

____

3. question

4. exclamatory sentence

Writers can improve their writing by carefully choosing simple sentence structures that begin with a specific subject and a strong verb. A strong verb shows clear action and is not a linking verb.

Original: There is a new patient in Room 15.

Revised: A new patient has been moved into Room 15.

Mr. Smith has been moved into Room 15.

Original: The child has a complaint about pain in his right side.

Revised: The child complains of pain in his right side.

EXERCISE 2-7: Use each of the following strong verbs in a sentence of your own. Refer to the unit glossary for definitions of these words.

1. intubate

2. elicit

3. palpate

4. incubate

5. ligate

UNIT PROOFREADING EXERCISES

Make the corrections by crossing out any errors or making edits by adding or removing words or punctuation.

A new medical devise has been approved by the Food and Drug Administration. Which is called The Merci Retriever. What device use? The device is made out of nitinol wire. Designed to rid the brain of blood clots. Blood clots debilitating and deadly.

Rewrite this passage here:

____

____

____

____

____

UNIT REVISION EXERCISES

Revise each sentence or sentence part to have a specific subject and a strong verb. You may need to add or remove words. Ensure that all sentences are complete.

1. There are plastic gloves to use for aseptic reasons.

____

____

2. There are the autopsy results.

____

____

3. It is estimated that the doctor will arrive by 9 o'clock.

____

____

4. Call me sometime today.

____

____

5. She has pain.

____

____

6. It is negative.

____

____

7. Cold compresses to the thigh.

____

____

8. If you stay fit.

____

____

9. There are too many guests in this room.

____

____

10. This stuff needs to be taken somewhere.

____

____

UNIT EXTENSIONS

1. Write a complete sentence that defines the word *suggestion*. Explain how this term *suggestion* could be taken in a positive as well as a negative way by a patient. Give an example of each interpretation.
2. Go to a medical website, such as www.webmd.com. Locate an article of interest and print it. Underline and label each subject and verb and label the independent and dependent clauses.
3. When you meet someone new or find someone you admire, what questions do you want to ask him or her? Write at least six questions.

UNIT 2 SELF-CHECK

Read each of the sentences below. Determine whether it is a independent clause (IC) or a dependent clause (DC).

______ **1.** When will the catheter be in place?

______ **2.** The technician prepared the slides for the supervisor to review.

______ **3.** If your asthma attack is triggered by cigarette smoke.

______ **4.** Because lowering your cholesterol may be difficult.

______ **5.** Your risk of a second stroke may be reduced by this medication.

Read each sentence below. Determine what essential sentence part is missing—subject (subj), verb (vb), or complete thought (ct)—or if the sentence is correct as written (ok). Write your answer on the line.

______ **6.** How we make healthcare coverage decisions.

______ **7.** Take antibiotics only as prescribed.

______ **8.** Many schools vision screening programs beginning in preschool years.

______ **9.** Also contribute to type 2 diabetes.

______ **10.** Eating healthfully and working out do not have to be difficult.

11–12. Read the boldfaced medical term and its definition. Then create a sentence of your own using this term.

edema: noun—a condition; an abnormal accumulation of fluids in the intercellular spaces of the body

____

____

throat culture: noun—a procedure; a bacteriological test used to identify throat pathogens, especially those associated with group A streptococci

____

____

UNIT 3

Expanding Sentence Basics

UNIT TERMS

Appositive phrase	A group of words that renames or describes the noun that precedes it; usually consists of adjectives and nouns
Article	*A, an, the;* used as adjectives
Clause	A group of words that includes a subject and a verb; may be a dependent clause or an independent clause
Compound sentence	A sentence that consists of two simple sentences, each of equal importance
Complex sentence	A sentence that consists of two clauses, an independent and a dependent clause, not of equal importance
Compound-complex sentence	A sentence that consists of three or more clauses: two independent clauses and at least one dependent clause
Conjunctive adverb	An adverb used to show a transition between two independent clauses
Coordinating conjunction	One of seven words in English *(and, but, for, nor, or, so, yet)* used to join equal grammatical units: word and word, phrase and phrase, or clause and clause
Dependent clause	A group of words that includes a subject and verb but does not express a complete thought; must attach to an independent clause to form a complete sentence
Independent clause	A group of words that includes a subject and verb and expresses a complete thought; can stand alone as a complete sentence
Main clause	Another name for an independent clause
Phrase	A group of words that lacks a subject, verb, or both
Subordinate clause	Another name for a dependent clause
Subordinating conjunction	Word used to join two clauses that are not equal in importance; shows the relationship of the sentence parts to each other

UNIT OBJECTIVES

Upon completion of this unit, the student will be able to

1. identify and draft appositive phrases
2. identify and draft compound sentences
3. identify and draft complex sentences
4. identify and draft compound-complex sentences
5. apply sentence order to ensure clarity in sentences

Glossary of Medical Terms

Term	Part of Speech	Definition
antibiotic	noun	a substance that destroys microorganisms
Braille	noun	a reading and writing system that allows the blind to see using touch
chicken pox	noun	a very contagious viral disease characterized by itchy red skin eruptions
contusion	noun	bruise
dysplasia	noun	abnormal development of tissue
ethnicity	noun	one's cultural background based on language, religion, or appearance
incontinence	noun	the inability to control urine, feces, or sperm because of a loss in muscle control
lipid	noun	a fat or fatty substance
narcolepsy	noun	a condition of chronic drowsiness and sleep
pediatrician	noun	a specialist in the treatment of children's diseases
ringworm	noun	a fungal infection of the skin
thrombosis	noun	the formation or development of a blood clot
tumor	noun	a swelling or enlargement; an abnormal growth

APPOSITIVE PHRASE

An appositive phrase consists of an article and/or an adjective and a noun or pronoun. An appositive phrase renames or describes further the noun that comes before it. There are also one-word appositives that include one-word definitions, names, or titles. These may or may not have commas separating them from the rest of the sentence. For example, *The patient's wife, Betty, is now here.*

Most appositive phrases are set off by commas if they occur in the middle of a sentence or by an initial comma if they are at the end of a sentence. The appositive phrase comes directly before or after the noun or pronoun it describes.

Noun Being Described	Comma	Renaming and Modifying Words (Adjectives)	Noun/Pronoun	Comma
surgeon	,	a well-known pediatric	cardiologist	,
carcinogen	,	high levels of	asbestos	,
diet	,	high-fiber, low-carbohydrate	meals	,
scalpel	,	a small straight-edged	knife	,

EXERCISE 3-1: Use this format to create appositive phrases of your own. Refer to the unit glossary for definitions of these words.

Noun Being Described	Comma	Modifying Words (Adjectives)	Noun/Pronoun	Comma
pediatrician				
ringworm				
contusion				
lipid				

To put this phrase into practice, one sentence pattern using appositive phrases is subject, comma, appositive phrase, comma, verb, and the rest of the sentence. This pattern is often used in healthcare to provide the definition of a term. For example:

> A basal cell carcinoma, *the most common type of skin cancer*, is often first discovered on the face, neck, or shoulder areas of the body.
>
> Senescence, *aging*, affects all parts of the human body. *(Note: no article or adjective is needed to modify aging.)*

Sometimes the appositive phrase is given at the end of the sentence. In this case, the pattern is subject, verb, noun, comma, appositive phrase. For example:

> Maria will schedule an endoscopic examination, *a viewing of the internal lining of her digestive tract.*
>
> Many young people have experience with herpes simplex, *a virus that causes blisters to form on the lips and inside the mouth.*

Using an appositive phrase is a simple and effective way to strengthen sentences by providing extra information with a few words. Textbooks in the healthcare fields often use this structure for providing definitions and supplying additional information. In classroom and report writing, an appositive phrase can clarify your knowledge of terms and conditions and eliminate the need for subordinate clauses, which tend to become wordy. Furthermore, the appositive phrase structure shows sophisticated conceptual thinking.

EXERCISE 3-2: Write simple sentences that include an appositive phrase. Follow each word with an appositive phrase that describes or clarifies the term. Refer to the unit glossary for definitions of these words. For example, <u>oncologist</u>:

> The <u>oncologist</u>, *a doctor specializing in treating cancers*, was well versed in a wide variety of treatment options.
>
> I need to see the oncologist, *a doctor specializing in treating cancers.*

1. tumor

2. Braille

3. ethnicity

4. chicken pox

5. thrombosis

Writers can shorten sentences with appositive phrases. Often an adjective clause may be rewritten as an appositive phrase. In doing so, the writer eliminates unnecessary words and allows punctuation to assist in expressing the thought. Look for describing clauses and phrases that modify the noun(s) and then make the appositive phrase where it most makes sense.

The doctor, who is a cardiologist, assisted the trauma team in the emergency room.

The doctor, a cardiologist, assisted the trauma team in the emergency room.

EXERCISE 3-3: Revise each sentence to include an appositive phrase.

1. Intimacy is the feeling of closeness with another person, and it is characterized by feelings of love, friendship, and companionship.

2. Medical asepsis refers to medical practices that reduce microorganisms and their transmission from one person to another and is referred to as clean technique.

3. Hand washing is central to isolation technique, and it is the single most important way to prevent the spread of infection.

4. The physical therapist does not work Monday; the physical therapist is a part-time student.

____

____

5. Presbyopia is due to a loss of elasticity in the eye's crystalline lens. Presbyopia is known as farsightedness.

____

____

THE COMPOUND SENTENCE

The compound sentence is a sentence that contains at least two independent or main clauses or simple sentences. Compound sentences do not include any dependent or subordinate clauses. Independent clauses must be joined in specific ways; three methods are used to join an independent clause to another independent clause:

1. with a coordinating conjunction (*and, but, for, nor, or, so yet*)
2. with a conjunctive adverb (*nevertheless, thus, however, consequently*)
3. with a semicolon (;)

These clauses can stand alone as simple sentences; however, they are joined to relate the ideas. Using compound sentences can help unify paragraphs and reduce choppy writing or writing that is hard to follow because there are too many short sentences.

The first pattern joins compound sentences with coordinating conjunctions. There are seven coordinating conjunctions in English; these are used to join equal grammatical units, like sentences. The seven coordinating conjunctions are *and, but, for, nor, or, so*, and *yet*. This sentence structure is particularly useful to show the relationship between main clauses. Careful selection of the coordinating conjunction will determine the relationship of one independent clause to the other.

Purpose or Function	Coordinating Conjunction to Select	Examples
To add additional information	and	*Muscle tissues push food through the stomach,* ***and*** *epithelial tissues use enzymes for absorption.*
To provide cause or reason and effect or result	for so	*Understanding cytology is important,* ***for*** *the process of disease begins at the cellular level.*
To show contrast or to contradict information	but yet	*Angina is not a disease,* ***but*** *it is a symptom of atherosclerosis.*
To present alternatives	or nor	*You may wait in the outpatient recovery area,* ***or*** *you may proceed to the general waiting area in the lobby.*

EXERCISE 3-4: Write compound sentences of your own in this pattern.

Independent Clause	,	Coordinating Conjunction	Independent Clause	.
		and		
		but		
		for (meaning: because)		
		nor		
		or		
		so		
		yet		

A second pattern for joining one independent clause to another independent clause is with a conjunctive adverb. This pattern is a bit more formal; however, it allows for more complex relationships between the two independent clauses.

Conjunctive adverbs are used to join some compound sentences because these adverbs assist the writer in showing the relationship between the sentence parts. The two sentences then have a relationship to each other, such as to provide additional information or to illustrate cause and effect. These relationships are provided by the conjunctive adverb. Review the purpose and functions of the conjunctive adverbs and the examples presented below.

Purpose or Function	Conjunctive Adverb to Select	Examples
To add additional information	in addition besides likewise moreover then	*Arteries carry blood from the heart to the rest of the body;* ***in addition,*** *they are the thickest vessels carrying blood under pressure.*
To provide cause or reason and effect or result	consequently hence accordingly thus therefore	*Irregular uterine bleeding between menstrual periods or after menopause may be symptomatic of some disease;* ***consequently,*** *early diagnosis and treatment should be sought.*
To show a contrast or to contradict information	however instead nevertheless	*The adrenal medulla is not an essential gland;* ***however,*** *it stimulates responses needed to handle emergencies.*
To present a time reference	meanwhile subsequently then thereafter	*The nervous system senses and interprets changes in internal and external environments;* ***then,*** *it coordinates an appropriate response to maintain the body's homeostasis.*
To indicate alternatives	otherwise	*You may go to the hospital pharmacy to pick up your prescription;* ***otherwise,*** *you may go to your local drugstore.*

EXERCISE 3-5: Write compound sentences of your own in this pattern.

Independent Clause	;	Conjunctive Adverb	,	Independent Clause	.

Conjunctive adverbs may occur within a simple sentence other than to join two main clauses. When this is the case, the conjunctive adverb is used for emphasis or to show a transition in thought. In this case, a comma, not a semicolon, is used to separate the conjunctive adverb from the sentence parts. The conjunctive adverb then functions as an interrupting phrase:

We will, however, meet in the family conference room.

Meanwhile, the patient should continue the drug regimen.

The third method of joining compound sentences is to join the two independent clauses with a semicolon. The semicolon serves as a signal that one independent clause has ended, and another is beginning.

Independent Clause	;	Independent Clause	.
The surgery proceeded well	;	*the patient is now in the recovery room*	.
Well-being varies among cultures	;	*diversity must be respected*	.
Appendicitis can be frightening	;	*medical help is needed immediately*	.
The insides of the artery walls are clogged	;	*the walls have thickened*	.

Notice that there is a relationship between the two clauses. When a writer uses the "independent clause; independent clause" construction, the purpose is to provide two equally powerful, yet related, statements. No transition words or conjunctions are used to join these two clauses. The brevity of the structure is its strongest asset.

EXERCISE 3-6: Write compound sentences of your own in this pattern.

Independent Clause	;	Independent Clause	.

Independent Clause	;	Independent Clause	.

THE COMPLEX SENTENCE

The complex sentence includes an independent clause and at least one dependent clause. The dependent clause, also called a subordinate clause, begins with a subordinating conjunction such as *because, although, since, after, when,* or *if.* Every complex sentence has at least one subordinate clause. Complex sentences are used to provide the reader with a hierarchy of information. The main clause is the most important sentence part, while the subordinate clause is secondary or supporting in nature. Complex sentences have several formats, presented below.

Understanding the specific purpose or function of subordinating conjunctions can assist the writer. Review the purpose, subordinating conjunction, and examples below.

Purpose or Function	Subordinating Conjunction to Select	Examples
To provide cause or reason and effect or result	because as since so that in order that	***Because*** *some organisms are so tiny, they are called microbes or microorganisms.*
To show a condition	if as if/even if unless as though/though although even though	***If*** *you help admit a patient, observe the patient carefully.* ***Although*** *all patients need privacy, patient safety is a priority.*
To present a time reference	after as as soon as before since while when	***When*** *illness occurs, it may limit a person's activities.* ***After*** *the pathogens enter the body, an infection can occur.*
To indicate a place	where wherever	***Where*** *moisture, light, nutrients, and warmth exist, pathogens can grow.*
To modify a person or thing	that who/whom which	*Membranes are epithelial tissues,* ***which*** *are supported by connective tissues.*

Complex sentences are written in three distinct patterns. The first pattern is dependent clause plus independent clause.

Dependent Clause	,	Independent Clause	.
When the cataracts were removed	,	the patient had clear vision	.
When people lose their mobility permanently	,	these patients need special care	.
If blood flow in the coronary arteries is decreased or diminished	,	myocardial damage may occur	.

A sentence that begins with a dependent clause is useful to draft when there is background information or minor detail that will add to the reader's understanding of the independent or main clause. Independent clauses contain the most important information and ideas. Dependent clauses offer an opportunity for the writer to add details and supporting ideas. When a sentence begins with a subordinate clause, a comma is placed at the end of the subordinate clause. The comma is a signal to the reader that the "big idea" is yet to be presented. By using this visual clue, the reader can quickly locate the most important ideas in sentences.

EXERCISE 3-7: The complex sentences below are partially written. Complete these complex sentences following the given pattern.

Dependent Clause	,	Independent Clause	.
When the flu season begins			
After the technician completes taking the X-rays			
		the dental assistant helped him	
As the surgical technician prepared the instruments			
		the doctor ordered a few more tests	

The second pattern of complex sentences places the independent or main clause first, and it is followed by the dependent or subordinate clause. A sentence beginning with an independent clause provides a strong structure of expression, for the main idea is provided before any details or other secondary information. This sentence pattern does not have a comma after the main clause and/or before the subordinate clause. A common error is the placement of a comma between the main clause and subordinate clause. This error can be avoided by careful proofreading.

Independent Clause	Dependent Clause	.
X-rays have shown the cause of his pain	so that he may seek treatment	.
A hernia is a protrusion or swelling of a tissue or an organ through a cavity wall	in which it is contained	.
Myocardial damage may occur	if blood flow in the coronary arteries is decreased or diminished	.

EXERCISE 3-8: The complex sentences below are partially written. Complete these complex sentences following the given pattern.

Independent Clause	Dependent Clause	.
The pharmacist can answer your prescription questions		
	since the nurse seemed very helpful	.
Certified nursing assistants provide for the basic daily care of the residents		
	if more recovery time is needed	.
Hospice is an organization designed to assist families with the care of their terminally ill loved ones		

The third and final pattern for complex sentences is started with a portion of the independent clause, the subordinate clause interrupts, and then the independent clause finishes.

Independent Clause Starts	,	Dependent Clause	,	Independent Clause Ends	.
The surgeon	,	who specializes in rhinoplasty	,	has an established practice in the medical center	.
Antitussives	,	which prevent or relieve coughing	,	act on the medullary center of the brain to inhibit the cough reflex	.
Code Red	,	which means there is a fire in the building	,	is part of the International Hospital Coding System	.

This sentence type uses the subordinate clause to provide additional supporting information for the subject. This information provides clarity or definition. A sentence that begins, is interrupted by a subordinate clause, and then finishes the main clause requires careful proofreading. A common error occurs when the writer creates a subject–verb agreement error by considering the interrupting clause as what determines the verb's form. The verb must agree with the subject of the sentence, not a noun within the subordinate clause. This type of error will be covered in Unit 5: Common Sentence Errors.

EXERCISE 3-9: The complex sentences below are partially written. Complete these complex sentences following the given pattern.

Independent Clause Starts	,	Dependent Clause	,	Independent Clause Ends	.
Some patients				do not rely on medication	.
		which the doctor prescribed			

(continued)

Independent Clause Starts	,	Dependent Clause	,	Independent Clause Ends	.
Diabetes				has two types, type 1 and type 2	.
		who was treated by this physician			

THE COMPOUND-COMPLEX SENTENCE

The compound-complex sentence consists of at least two independent clauses and at least one dependent or subordinate clause. This type of structure is used to present fairly complex ideas and should be used infrequently. These sentences tend to become wordy, so this construction sometimes makes the content difficult to understand. Therefore, one should use compound-complex sentences sparingly.

Patterns for compound-complex sentences vary but essentially include any combination of compound sentence patterns and complex sentence patterns. Compound-complex sentences must have at least three distinct clauses: two independent clauses and at least one subordinate clause. Some examples are provided below.

Independent Clause	,	Coordinating Conjunction	Independent Clause	Subordinate Clause	.
Maslow's theory puts human development on a hierarchy of importance	,	and	physical needs must be met	before any other need can be dealt with	.
The patient needs to see a specialist	,	but	he is unsure	whom he should contact	.

Two other ways to organize a compound-complex sentence are given below.

Dependent Clause	,	Independent Clause	;	Conjunctive Adverb	,	Independent Clause	.
As people age	,	they seem to enjoy reminiscing	;	however	,	remembering past events may make them sad at times	.
Since the patient needs to see a specialist	,	our office will contact the doctor's office	;	however	,	the patient must arrange his own transportation to the medical appointment	.
If you consider the health risks of unprotected sex	,	you will avoid risky behavior	;			you will thus avoid certain communicable diseases	.

Independent Clause	,	Dependent Clause	, or ;	Independent Clause	.
A patient may seek a specialist	,	who is well known in a medical field	,	he may request a second opinion about a procedure	.
This prescription is expensive	,	which is unfortunate	;	sometimes there are no options for using generics to reduce the cost of medicine	.
Diabetes has two types, type 1 and type 2	,	which create medical challenges for an individual	,	but good documentation and lifestyle management can help manage the disease	.

EXERCISE 3-10: Review the compound-complex sentence patterns. Write four sentences of your own using this sentence type. Use appropriate medical terminology and the context of healthcare for your subject matter. Refer to the unit glossary for possible words to use in your sentences.

1. ______________________________
   ____
2. ______________________________
   ____
3. ______________________________
   ____
4. ______________________________
   ____

These basic sentence structures appear throughout healthcare texts. By understanding these structures and the strengths of each sentence type, writers can enhance their sentence-writing techniques.

PHRASE VERSUS CLAUSE

Knowing the difference between a phrase and a clause is important because it allows the writer to make choices in selecting specific sentence structures. Often, the writer is limited in time, words, or space; therefore, the writer may choose a phrase over a clause, as in the following example:

> The patient suffers from conjunctivitis, *an inflammation of the delicate membrane lining the inside of the eyelid and surface of the eye.* (phrase)
>
> The patient suffers from conjunctivitis, *which is an inflammation of the delicate membrane lining the inside of the eyelid and surface of the eye.* (clause)
>
> Photophobia, *the inability to tolerate bright lights,* is one of the symptoms of meningitis. (phrase)

Photophobia, *which is the inability to tolerate bright lights*, is one of the symptoms of meningitis. (clause)

Clauses usually lengthen the sentences and are introduced by subordinating conjunctions. Thus, phrases minimize the number of words in a sentence, and they often provide for powerful sentences, sentences with a lot of information and fewer words.

EXERCISE 3-11: Shorten these sentences by making the clauses into phrases.

1. The presence of group A streptococci, which are bacteriological throat pathogens, needs to be confirmed.

____

____

2. Doctors who are called gerontologists diagnose and treat aging patients.

____

____

3. A new device that is referred to as the Merci Retriever can remove blood clots from the brain.

____

____

4. West Nile virus, which is a mosquito-borne virus, appears to be on the rise in the western portions of the United States.

____

____

SENTENCE ORDER

Sentence order provides a hierarchy for emphasis. We usually place the most important idea at the beginning of a sentence. The subject or topic usually is provided before other details. Note that when the main idea is not presented first, then the first phrase or clause is usually separated from the main idea by some form of punctuation.

EXERCISE 3-12: Underline the main idea in the sentences below.

1. When your doctor is off duty, other doctors are designated to provide for your care.

2. Healthcare agencies developed policies that describe the guidelines under which patients may read their records.

3. A law is an established and enforced rule of conduct that is intended to protect the rights of people.

4. An anecdotal note is a written record that presents the facts of a specific event.

5. Military time is a method of expressing time that uses a different four-digit number for each of the day's hours and minutes.

UNIT PROOFREADING EXERCISES

Read the paragraph below. Edit the sentences for correct sentence punctuation. Add or delete punctuation as needed.

Many young people are concerned about their body images. They do not want to be overweight they do not want to be too tall or too short. Peer pressure is very strong during the adolescent period. Any change in a body, is noticed. Sometimes teens are teased so they feel even more self-conscious. These issues about body image are reinforced by the media which plays advertisements showing skinny bodies, lots of skin; and a carefree lifestyle. It is easy to understand. Many youth feel ashamed by their changing bodies and weight gain. During this time it is important that parents ensure a proper diet, plenty of exercise, and positive mentoring of friends and family.

UNIT REVISION EXERCISES

Change these clauses into appositive phrases.

1. The surgeon, who is a pediatric dermatologist, suggested that we wait until Brittany is past her growth spurts before we attempt surgery.

____

____

2. The medicine, which is called Bactrim Suspension, is commonly used for ear infections in children.

____

____

3. The practice moved to a new building, which is called the Highway Medical Center.

____

____

4. Some herbal remedies, which may be popular but untested medicines, can be dangerous if the dosing is not controlled.

____

____

5. Brown rice, which is a high-fiber food, is popular with many people who are watching their intake of carbohydrates.

Make these compound-complex sentences into two shorter sentences.

6. The budget needs to cover needed equipment; the medical staff believes that a new autoclave will ensure instrument sterilization in a shorter amount of time and at a lower cost.

7. The medicine cart that needs to be repaired is missing a wheel part, so the cart always travels at an angle instead of in a straight line.

8. The floor volunteers have done a nice job of ensuring that patients have reading materials; in addition, they are providing opportunities for light discussion, which is so important for those patients who have been in the hospital a long time.

UNIT EXTENSIONS

1. Locate a journal article in your field of interest. Copy the article. Tally the different types of sentences.

Sentence Type	Number located in the article
Simple	
Compound	
Complex	
Compound-Complex	

2. Write a paragraph about head lice. Use appropriate vocabulary to discuss this topic. Perform a readability test by using the tools on the computer to calculate the reading level of your passage. Select the paragraph. In Microsoft Word, under the Tools menu, select Spelling and Grammar; and under Options, click on Readability. Then check the document and review the reading level. When creating a document for the public and for educational purposes, the Flesch-Kincaid readability index should be between Grade 5 and Grade 7 to ensure comprehension by the most readers.

3. Develop a graphic that illustrates the cycle of a disease. Some topics might include head lice, hepatitis, AIDS, influenza, or diabetes. Write several sentences to summarize the main idea of the graphic.

UNIT 3 SELF-CHECK

Use the sentences to create a new sentence in the pattern requested.

1. The doctor specializes in pediatric brain surgeries. The doctor is a pediatric neurologist. (Combine to form a simple sentence that includes an appositive phrase.)

____

____

2. People are living longer. Blood pressure tends to rise with age. It also rises with weight gain or obesity. (Combine to form a compound sentence that is joined with *and*.)

____

____

3. A new test for cholesterol is being researched. This test allows the blood to be tested any time. The current test requires the patient to fast for 12 hours prior to the test. (Combine to form a compound-complex sentence.)

____

____

4. Research has shown a link between soft drinks and type 2 diabetes. We need to encourage alternatives to sugary beverages for our children. (Combine to form a complex sentence.)

____

____

Choose from these categories to label each sentence or sentence part below:

- Appositive phrase
- Coordinating conjunction
- Conjunctive adverb
- Subordinating conjunction
- Fragment
- Simple sentence
- Compound sentence
- Complex sentence

5. ____________________ ; therefore,

6. ____________________ The call for type O blood has been placed.

7. ____________________ although

8. ____________________ The pharmacy is about to close; the pharmacist will still assist you.

9. ____________________ Since the beginning of the clinic construction

10. ____________________ , a registered nurse,

11. ____________________ or

12. ____________________ While the baby is resting, you need to call your insurance provider.

UNIT 4

Effective Sentence Structures

UNIT TERMS

Active voice	The subject doing the verb's action
Jargon	Overly technical language
Passive voice	The subject receiving the verb's action
Slang	Informal word or phrase choices
Voice	Verbs have two voices, active and passive.

UNIT OBJECTIVES

Upon completion of this unit, the student will be able to

1. identify active and passive voice in sentences
2. revise passive sentences to become active sentences
3. identify effective sentence choice
4. revise *it is* and *there are* sentence starters
5. use the comma correctly in sentences
6. use the semicolon correctly in sentences
7. use the colon correctly in sentences
8. use the hyphen correctly in sentences
9. revise sentences to ensure proper punctuation
10. choose effective vocabulary for healthcare writing

Glossary of Medical Terms

Term	Part of Speech	Definition
acute	adjective	severe, sharp, occurring quickly
autonomic system	noun	the part of the nervous system that controls involuntary body functions
bactericide	noun	an agent that destroys bacteria
catheter	noun	a tube passed through the body to remove fluids
diarrhea	noun	loose, fluid, or unformed bowel movements or stools
dietitian	noun	a specialist trained in the area of nutrition

flossing	noun	the act of cleaning by rubbing floss or thread between the teeth to remove plaque or food
hypochondriac	noun	a person who has an abnormal fear of disease or illness
jaundice	noun	a condition of excess bilirubin in the blood; characterized by yellowing skin, whites of eyes, and mucous membranes
parasympathetic	adjective	one part of the autonomic nervous system
physical therapist	noun	a specialist trained in the treatment of restorative care
prognosis	noun	an opinion on the course of a disease or illness
restorative	adjective	describes returning something to its previous state or condition; to restore
rounds	noun	a scheduled duty performed by the healthcare professional to check on the progress and condition of hospital patients
soluble	adjective	dissolvable
sympathetic	adjective	one part of the autonomic nervous system

SENTENCES IN ACTIVE AND PASSIVE VOICE

Verbs have two voices, active and passive. A sentence written in the active voice has the subject doing the verb's action. A sentence written in the passive voice has the subject receiving the verb's action or not personally doing the verb's action.

Healthcare students need to understand the difference between the active and passive voice for two reasons. First of all, many textbooks use passive structures to discuss medical procedures. Second, writers should use the active voice because it is easier to understand, and this structure is more focused. In other words, the reader wants to know who did what. The passive voice tends to lack clarity and is a less efficient structure.

Voice	Example	Explanation
Active	The nurse prepared the medications for the morning rounds.	The nurse is the subject, and the nurse does the action—*prepare.*
Passive	The medications for the morning rounds were prepared by the nurse.	The medication is the subject, and it receives the action of *prepared* passively.
Passive	The medications for the morning rounds were prepared.	The medication is the subject and it receives the action of *prepared.*
Active	The dental assistant positioned the examination chair.	The dental assistant is the subject and does the action—*positioned.*
Passive	The chair was positioned by the dental assistant.	The chair is the subject, and it receives the action of *positioned.*

Sometimes the passive voice includes who is doing the action, and sometimes it does not. There are times that it is not necessary to know specifically who is doing the verb's action. For example, *Your insurance claim was forwarded to your provider.* In this case, we do not need to know that Shelly Fairfield forwarded the insurance claim. Companies and governmental agencies often use this type of communication.

Consider for a moment government policies or workplace safety posters:

New safety procedures are in place for handling needles.

New patients' rights policies are in place in this hospital.

These regulations are set by OSHA.

Usually, the reader is not really concerned who made these policies or rules, so it is appropriate that these are written in the passive voice.

The passive voice is used for three specific purposes:

1. to express an action, but not reveal the actor

   The patient complaint was filed with the hospital administrator.
   Your outstanding bill was given to a collection agency.

2. to express an action, but the actor is unknown

   The room preparation was completed thirty minutes ago.
   The dumpster has been remodeled with a safety cover.

3. to focus the reader on the action, not the actor

   Polio was considered a prominent disease in the early 1900s.
   Auto accidents are considered a leading cause of teen injuries.

EXERCISE 4-1: Read the sentences below and indicate whether each is written in the active or passive voice.

Sentences for Review	Voice of Verb: Active or Passive
The new procedure is being reviewed by the hospital board.	
Nurses attended a training session in the conference room.	
A mistake was made in the documentation of this case.	
The reference manuals were placed in the staff work room.	
The certified nursing assistants assisted the nursing staff at the healthcare fair.	

EXERCISE 4-2: Provide the active voice for each of the sentences below.

Sentence Written in Passive Voice	Revision in Active Voice
The nurse was assigned a new shift.	
The outdated medical records were shredded.	
The extraction was done in the dentist's office.	
The bandage was removed and discarded.	
Blood pressure readings were taken twice a day.	

AVOIDING *IT* AND *THERE* AS SENTENCE STARTERS

In keeping with strong and effective communication, writers need to keep their sentence starters focused on who is doing the verb's action. Oral communication and written communication vary a great deal. Sometimes writers rely on the patterns of oral communication rather than effective written structures. One example of oral communication is the use of *it is, there is,* or *there are* structures. To avoid weak sentence starters, *it is* and *there is/are* should be avoided. *It* is a pronoun, and it replaces a noun; however, it is not specific. *There* is an adverb and cannot be a subject.

Ineffective Sentence Starters	Revised Sentence Starters
It is the patient's request to seek a second opinion.	The patient requests a second opinion.
It is necessary to make changes in your healthcare coverage.	Your healthcare coverage needs changing.
There was nothing for the nurses to do except make the patient comfortable.	The nurses made the patient comfortable.
There were too many unanswered questions about the new procedure.	Too many unanswered questions remain about the new procedure.

The revised sentence starters illustrate the change made from ineffective sentence starters to effective sentence starters. By using specific subjects, the reader understands up front who is doing the verb's action. This revision helps keep the sentences focused.

EXERCISE 4-3: Make the revision to rid the sentence of ineffective starters.

Ineffective Sentence Starters	Revised Sentence Starters
There were last-minute arrangements that needed to be made prior to patient's admission to the residential center.	
It is necessary for some medical staff to have beepers in this wing of the hospital.	
There is a requirement that you submit to a urinalysis for drug testing prior to employment.	
It is our mission to serve all patients who request medical care and family counseling.	
It is advised that the patient should not participate in vigorous activity.	

USING COMMAS (,)

Punctuation is important in writing. We use pauses in our natural speech patterns when we speak; however, in writing we cannot pause, so we use commas. Commas help the reader by providing divisions between words, thoughts, and expressions.

Rules for Commas with Clauses	Examples
Use a comma followed by a coordinating conjunction (*and, but, for, or, nor, yet, so*) to separate two main clauses.	The patient is in the lounge waiting for the family counselor, and he is on time for his appointment.
Use a comma to separate an initial dependent clause from an independent clause.	Whenever she felt nervous, she used deep breathing exercises to calm herself.

Use a comma before a clause that begins with *which*. *Which* introduces a clause that provides extra information, so it is separated by one or more commas, depending on its location in a sentence.	The health club, which specializes in women's health, was a feature of the show. The show featured a health club, which specializes in women's health.

Exercise 4-4: Write one sentence for each pattern given below.

Rules for Commas with Clauses	Examples
Use a comma followed by a coordinating conjunction *(and, but, for, or, nor, yet, so)* to separate two main clauses.	
Use a comma to separate an initial dependent clause from an independent clause.	
Use a comma before a clause that begins with *which*. *Which* introduces a clause that provides extra information, so it is separated by one or more commas, depending on its location in a sentence.	

In addition, commas are used to set off introductory items in sentences. The rules for using commas after initial structures are given below.

Rules for Commas with Words and Phrases	Examples
Use a comma for a series.	The patients were here to see the doctor, the nurse, and the physical therapist.
Use a comma after introductory comments such as *Well, Oh, Yes,* or *No.*	Yes, I am applying for the residency at the Valley Hospital.
Use a comma after introductory phrases.	To be healthy, Bob avoided sweets. Looking in the mirror, Sam felt the dental surgery was a success. In the morning, the patient will have the catheter removed.
Use a comma between multiple adjectives before a noun.	The confident, self-reliant healthcare student searched for errors as he proofread his report.
Use a comma after a person's name and before a title.	Ms. Sally Nether, RN, PA, will answer any questions you might have.
Use commas around appositive phrases if they are midsentence and before a final appositive phrase in a sentence.	The medical team leader, Dr. Arra Smith, is meeting with the family this morning. I would like to present my research paper, "A Link Between Diet and Disease."

Exercise 4-5: Write one sentence for each pattern given below.

Rules for Commas with Words and Phrases	Examples
Use a comma for a series.	
Use a comma after introductory comments such as *Well, Oh, Yes,* or *No.*	

(continued)

Rules for Commas with Words and Phrases	Examples
Use a comma after introductory phrases.	
Use a comma between multiple adjectives before a noun.	
Use a comma after a person's name and before a title.	
Use commas around appositive phrases if they are midsentence and before a final appositive phrase in a sentence.	

USING SEMICOLONS, COLONS, AND HYPHENS

Punctuation can assist you in ensuring that the reader can easily understand your writing. Using semicolons, colons, and hyphens adds style to basic sentence structure and gives you a choice of organizational pattern.

SEMICOLON (;)

A semicolon is a more formal punctuation mark than a comma. Semicolons separate two independent clauses or items in a series that also include commas. In this case, the semicolon helps keep the segments of a list distinctly separated. Three rules for using semicolons are given below.

Rules for Using Semicolons	Examples
Use a semicolon to separate two independent clauses.	Computers make billing inquiries easy to verify; medical billers can monitor activity and access account information from any workstation.
Use a semicolon with a conjunctive adverb and a comma to separate two independent clauses.	Harriet needed a blood transfusion; therefore, we stayed in the recovery center a bit longer than expected.
Use a semicolon to separate items in a series that has internal commas.	Merci of Life Centers will be set up in Rome, Italy; Houston, Texas; Los Angeles, California; and New York, New York.

EXERCISE 4-6: Write one sentence for each pattern given below.

Rules for Using Semicolons	Examples
Use a semicolon to separate two independent clauses.	
Use a semicolon with a conjunctive adverb and a comma to separate two independent clauses.	
Use a semicolon to separate items in a series that has internal commas.	

COLON (:)

A colon is most often used to indicate a list or series. Do not use words like *such as* or *like* with a colon. An independent clause usually precedes a colon. The rules and situations for using colons are given below.

Rules for Using Colons	Examples
Use a colon preceding a list or series that is not introduced by a verb.	The utility cart needs the following: sheets, pillow slips, washcloths, toilet paper, bactericide, and liquid soap.
Use a colon to distinguish hours from minutes in time.	5:30 P.M. or 9:00 A.M.
Use a colon after a formal salutation in a business letter.	Dear Dr. Barry Brown:
Use a colon to emphasize a word, phrase, clause, or sentence that explains or adds impact to the main clause.	The dentist gave her one option: Remove the decayed tooth
Use a colon to distinguish between a title and subtitle, volume and page, or chapter and verse.	The Medical Assistant: Self-Care Encyclopedia Medica III: 223 Psalm 23:1–4
Use a colon to introduce a quotation, question, or sentence.	The doctor told the family: "Decisions need to be made regarding Helen's care."

EXERCISE 4-7: Write one sentence for each pattern given below.

Rules for Using Colons	Examples
Use a colon preceding a list or series that is not introduced by a verb.	
Use a colon to distinguish hours from minutes in time.	
Use a colon after a formal salutation in a business letter.	
Use a colon to emphasize a word, phrase, clause, or sentence that explains or adds impact to the main clause.	
Use a colon to distinguish between a title and subtitle, volume and page, or chapter and verse.	
Use a colon to introduce a quotation, question, or sentence.	

HYPHEN (-)

A hyphen is used between the parts of words that must be divided at the end of a line and between some compound words.

Rules for Using Hyphens	Examples
Use a hyphen for compound adjectives that modify one word, such as family-oriented practice, one-way street, one-in-ten chance.	Our new patient is a middle-aged person who wants to begin an exercise program.
Use a hyphen for writing out compound numbers between 21 and 99, such as twenty-one or fifty-five.	Seventy-three individuals will receive notices of the next healthcare fair.
Use a hyphen with fractions, such as two-thirds or one-fourth.	One-third of the filing work is to be completed by the medical receptionist today.
Use a hyphen to join certain prefixes and roots such as *self-*, *all-*, and *ex-*. Refer to a dictionary if unsure.	The child has a great deal of self-control.
Use a hyphen to divide a word at its syllable division point at the end of a line.	The team meeting will be held to have a discussion about sharing work-load this week.

EXERCISE 4-8: Write one sentence for each pattern given below.

Rules for Using Hyphens	Examples
Use a hyphen for compound adjectives that modify one word, such as family-oriented practice, one-way street, one-in-ten chance.	
Use a hyphen for writing out compound numbers between 21 and 99, such as twenty-one or fifty-five.	
Use a hyphen with fractions, such as two-thirds or one-fourth.	
Use a hyphen to join certain prefixes and roots such as *self-*, *all-*, and *ex-*. Refer to a dictionary if unsure.	
Use a hyphen to divide a word at its syllable division point at the end of a line.	

CHOOSING EFFECTIVE VOCABULARY

One strategy to assist you in writing more specific sentences is to use medical terms and specific phrases used in the healthcare field. One important tool is a medical dictionary. Many medical dictionaries are available for writers. These are useful because they include the term, its pronunciation, diagrams if applicable, and related terms. Interestingly, these types of dictionaries use subheadings to further explain the basic terms: nursing diagnosis, cautions, nursing implications, etiology, prognosis, first aid, systems, treatment, and so on. In addition, the appendices of these dictionaries contain a wealth of information: abbreviations, list of specialties, dietary allowances, medical emergency information, prefixes, suffixes, root words, prescription terms, and diagnostic-related information.

Writers cannot expect to have a background in medical terminology merely because they are interested in healthcare. Time is needed to learn how to use the terms properly. However, some guidelines do exist to help beginning writers:

1. When you are reading a textbook or journal article about healthcare, focus on the terms used and the style of language. When you write about that chapter or article, try to use the medical terms and the style.
2. Keep a notebook or index cards with specific medical terms you are learning. Note their part of speech and any related words associated with the term. By learning words in "families" or groups, writers can associate meanings more easily.
3. Avoid jargon or slang. Many times patients will speak to you in rather informal terms because that is their experience. Your choice of terms will be clinical, while theirs may be emotional or physical. Typically, the goal is not to intimidate a patient with terms that he or she does not understand. The healthcare worker must adapt his or her language patterns to the patient to ensure professional communication.
4. Avoid overwriting or writing to impress. Sometimes writers use more technical terminology that is needed, and the message is difficult to understand. A good rule of thumb is to keep the message simple and to the point. Use specific words.
5. Avoid sentence starters such as *I think, personally, it is my opinion, I believe that.* Avoid these sentence starters because whatever you write is your opinion unless it is documented from another source.

Read the examples of ineffective vocabulary and the revisions below. The revisions are more directed and specific.

Examples of Ineffective Vocabulary	Revisions
It is my opinion that the procedure needs further testing to ensure that it is safe.	The procedure needs further safety testing.
He has a lot of anger.	His anger results from his prognosis and his inability to control his health.
She has nasty diarrhea.	She has acute diarrhea.
Your food needs to be varied.	Your diet needs to be balanced across the food groups.
The baby is yellow.	The baby has jaundice.

EXERCISE 4-9: Revise each sentence, providing effective vocabulary.

Examples of Ineffective Vocabulary	Revisions
The man is all scratched up.	
The knife wound butchered him like a chicken on the cutting block.	

(continued)

Examples of Ineffective Vocabulary	Revisions
I am happy.	
I believe that she feels sad about the death of her mama.	
She has a big black splotch on her leg.	

UNIT PROOFREADING EXERCISES

Read the following passage. Then neatly cross out the errors and make the changes necessary for clear communication.

Sumamry of the Patient's Writes

The american hospital association published The Patient's Bill of Rights in 1973. In my opinion, the purpose of this document focuses on the responsible of the hospitals and the patients. The objective is to increase communication and collaboration between these parties. The patient is supposed to get consideration and respect while receiving care; true and under-standable information about his or her condition, privacy and confidentiality and a response to treatment request. The patient's responsibilities include giving up any information that might effect his or her treatment, insurance information, and pertinent lifestyle information. The goal is to ensure that both the hospital and the patient get the necessary information to provide and receive the best care possible.

UNIT REVISION EXERCISES

Revise these sentences to ensure more specific expression.

1. For this procedure, there are eight steps that must be carried out.

____

2. It is assumed that this individual is a hypochondriac.

____

3. There is a dental assistant who tells everybody how important brushing and flossing are to do.

____

____

Revise the following sentences to include semicolons, colons, commas, and hyphens.

4. The patient needs to ingest fat soluble vitamins.

____

5. The autonomic system has two divisions the sympathetic and the parasympathetic.

____

6. Fellow healthcare professionals tonight my talk will cover breast research.

____

7. An injured man came into the emergency entrance; his wound was v shaped.

____

8. The diet was rich in calcium potassium minerals and folic acid.

____

9. Dietitians are hired to ensure proper and restorative nutritional intake long term care residents need someone to assist them to ensure they have a balanced diet.

____

Change this sentence from passive to active.

10. The surgical procedure was completed with the use of a tiny laser.

____

UNIT EXTENSIONS

1. A patient's insurance company has denied a payment on an invoice. Draft a sentence that politely tells the patient that the bill is now his or her responsibility to pay.
2. Write a note specifically thanking a caregiver for excellent care. Be clear what the care was and what your heartfelt feelings are.
3. Do a web search on childhood vaccinations. Write sentences detailing the immunizations and their expected benefits. Use specific medical terminology.

UNIT 4 SELF-CHECK

Mark the sentences as correct or rewrite, making the changes as needed.

1. Three categories of community agencies exist to provide numerous patient services; private, governmental, and nonprofit.

____

____

2. The seven-teen page document belongs to Dr. Fields.

____

____

3. He is part of a family oriented dental practice.

4. The plan is to operate however if the tests come back with new information that plan can change.

Rewrite as active sentences:

5. The doctor was asked to explain his decision to the committee.

6. The old fabric chairs in the sun room were recycled.

7. The excision was done in the outpatient surgery wing of the hospital.

8. The tumor was removed and sent to the lab.

Revise each sentence to ensure effective communication:

9. I think that the kid was all banged up.

10. It is my opinion that the insurance is the best thing since sliced bread.

Look at the medical terminology in boldface below. Write a sentence of your own using the terms.

lymphoidectomy (*noun*) surgical removal of lymphoid tissue

11. ______

incise (*verb*) to make a cut into; to cut with a sharp instrument

12. ______

UNIT 5

Common Sentence Errors

UNIT TERMS

Agreement	The matching of number and gender of words
Antecedent	A word that is referred to by another
Comma splice	Two independent clauses joined by only a comma
Dangling modifier	A word group that is not modifying the intended term
Modifier	A word or group of words that describes or explains another term
Parallel structure	Similar elements that are coordinated and equal in form
Past participle	Verb ending in *–ed, –en*, or irregular spelling
Run-on sentence	Two independent clauses that are not joined correctly
Tense	The time an action takes place; shown by verbs

UNIT OBJECTIVES

Upon completion of this unit, the student will be able to

1. recognize common types of sentence errors

2. correct common sentence errors

3. draft sentences in parallel structure

4. revise sentences with tense errors

Glossary of Medical Terms

Term	Part of Speech	Definition
anatomy	noun	the structure of an organism
chemotherapy	noun	the use of chemicals to destroy disease-causing microorganisms
dermatologist	noun	a specialist in the treatment and prevention of skin disease
excise	verb	to remove; to cut out
gauze	noun	a light woven fabric used in medical supplies such as bandages and sponges
leishmania	noun	a parasitic disease caused by bites of female sandflies
lumbar	adjective	describes a part of the back; the area between the thorax and pelvis
massage	verb, noun	manipulation, rubbing, kneading, and pressure used on the body
microbiology	noun	the study of microorganisms
microorganisms	noun	minute living bodies such as bacteria or protozoa

MRI	noun	magnetic resonance imaging; a type of diagnostic radiography
physiology	noun	the science of the functions of living organisms and their parts
stem cell	noun	a hemocytoblast or cell found in bone marrow and lymphatic tissue that generates blood cells
stroke	noun	a sudden loss of consciousness followed by paralysis caused by thrombosis or hemorrhage

SUBJECT–VERB ERRORS

Subjects and verbs must agree in number (singular and plural) and person (first, second, third). To agree in number, the writer must match the subject in number with the correct verb form:

> He needs to see his doctor immediately.
>
> The interns were restless as they waited for their shift supervisor.

Most writers correctly match subject and verbs in these types of sentences. The errors occur in more complex sentence structures. To ensure proper agreement, follow these steps:

1. Locate the verb.
2. Locate the subject and determine if it is singular or plural.
3. Ensure the verb matches the subject in number and person.

For example:

There is junk food and sodas filling his refrigerator.

1. Locate the verb (*is*).
2. Locate the subject and determine if it is singular or plural (*junk food and sodas* = plural).
3. Ensure the verb matches the subject in number and person (change verb to *are*): *There are junk food and sodas filling his refrigerator.*

There are some guidelines to help determine subject–verb agreement. These are listed below.

Guidelines for Subject–Verb Agreement	Example
In the present tense, the singular subjects of *he, she, person, one,* and the like have a verb that ends in −*s*. Singular subjects of *I* and *you* take irregular forms of the verb or do not have a −*s*. Plural subjects agree with verbs that do not end in −*s*.	The volunteer *rubs* the patient's back to relax him. Nurses *work* hard to ensure good care. I *am* in the healthcare field. He *works* four 10-hour shifts at the clinic. You *need* to report to the head nurse.

Some indefinite pronoun subjects have verbs that end in *–s* (*one, everybody, someone, each, kind, either, neither, sort, type, anything*, and the like).	Everyone *has gathered* for the medical consultation. This sort of precaution *is* usual. Neither of the doctors *is* available.
Some plural pronoun subjects have verbs that do not end in *–s* (*lots, many, kinds, both, several*, and the like).	Both of the day surgery centers *are closing* for the long weekend.
When a subject is followed by a prepositional phrase, use the subject to determine the verb. A common error is to use the noun in the prepositional phrase.	Bob, along with the other children, *has* an appointment with the dentist this morning. His nurse, together with the doctor, *is* at lunch.
Some pronoun subjects *(all, none, some)* can have singular or plural verbs.	None of the therapists *is* working Sunday. None of the prescriptions *are* filled yet.
That, which, and *who* as subjects can either have a verb or verb + *s*. Note: These subjects often occur in adjective or describing clauses.	The doctors who *respond* are willing to learn the new technique in Dallas. The medical assistant who *arrives* on time is appreciated.
Units of measure, money, and time take verbs that end in *–s*.	One hundred dollars *seems* like a lot for a medical consultation. Fifty pounds *is* a lot to lose that quickly.
Some diseases or subjects of study are singular nouns ending in *–s*, and these take verbs that end in *–s* (*measles, diabetes, rickets, mathematics, physics*, and the like).	Measles *is* a disease that has been controlled by vaccination programs. Physics *plays* a role in balance and physical therapy.
Singular nouns joined by *or* or *nor* take verbs that end in *–s*.	The nurse or the certified nursing assistant *is* available to help move the patient.
If the plural and singular nouns are joined by *or* or *nor*, then the noun closest to the verb determines if the verb does or does not end in *–s*.	The nurse or her assistants are available to assist in transferring the patient. Neither the residents nor the administrator *knows* the answer to that question.

EXERCISE 5-1: Write *S* for singular or *P* for plural in the blank to the right of each word or word group.

1. phlebotomist ____________
2. a doctor who ____________
3. any kind ____________
4. somebody ____________
5. Sal, along with the boys ____________
6. all of the staff ____________
7. ten pounds ____________
8. a few thermometers ____________
9. therapy ____________
10. bacterium ____________

Exercise 5-2: Underline the verb that agrees with the subject.

1. Economics (do, does) influence healthcare decisions.
2. There (is, are) no staff member available to assist the patient.
3. Either the parent or the guardian (need, needs) to authorize this procedure.
4. Training and experience (contribute, contributes) to the excellence of Bella Hospital.
5. Each of you (have, has) a task to accomplish in Room 523.
6. Without computers, the medical receptionists (do, does) not have access to your insurance records.
7. The medical team (is, are) waiting for the lab results.
8. In the newborn area, registered nurses (gather, gathers) to view the twins.
9. Neither the child nor the parents (was, were) feeling well.
10. The doctor, along with his assistants, (intend, intends) to operate to remove the tumor.

Exercise 5-3: Complete the sentences below.

1. Either the patients or the nurse ______________________________
____
2. The staff ______________________________________
____
3. Every one of the ________________________________
____
4. The nurse, together with the medical assistants, _____________
____
5. Dental assistants and dental hygienists _________________
____

PRONOUN–ANTECEDENT AGREEMENT ERRORS

A pronoun must refer to a specific noun to make sense. This noun is called the antecedent. When a writer has a noun and the pronoun following that noun changes person or number, this is called an error in pronoun–antecedent agreement.

Guidelines for Pronoun–Antecedent Agreement	Example
Use singular pronouns *(he, she, it, his, him, her, hers)* to agree with a singular noun or pronoun.	The doctor is calling *her* assistant. Bertha sees *her* aide, and *she* needs to speak with him.

Use plural pronouns *(they, them,* and *theirs)* to agree with a plural noun or pronoun.	Long term residents require *their* own rooms. The staff members are concerned; *they* will assist the family in helping the patient with his goals.
Singular indefinite pronouns (*anything, no one, each, sort, type, somebody, neither, either, kind, each,* and the like) require singular pronouns in formal grammar.	Neither family member left *his* name. *It* is the kind of illness that is treatable.
In sentences that include a *neither–nor* or *either–or* construction, the pronoun should match the nouns with the singular or plural forms. If the nouns differ, then the pronoun will agree with the subject closest to the pronoun.	Neither the bandage nor the wrap *is* able to be secured on that wound. Either the computers or the software *needs* to be updated in the health clinic.

EXERCISE 5-4: Write the pronoun in the blank to the right of each word or word group.

1. phlebotomist ____________
2. Mr. Edward Smithers ____________
3. anyone ____________
4. somebody ____________
5. Sally, along with the boys____________
6. all of the instruments ____________
7. ten pounds ____________
8. a few thermometers ____________
9. therapy ____________
10. specimen slides ____________

EXERCISE 5-5: Underline the pronoun that agrees with its antecedent.

1. The cost of care may make a person decide (he, they) cannot afford the elective surgery.
2. Each of the female patients needs to have (her, their) own prenatal file.
3. Either the parent or the guardian needs to authorize this claim for (his, their) child.
4. Training is important for all new employees; (he, it, they) need to understand our policies and procedures.
5. How does the hospital handle (his, its) patients?
6. The administrator asked all of (we, us) to outline solutions to assist in the conflict resolution.
7. The medical laboratory is fully staffed; (their, its) employees are now in training.

8. The decision about elective care is between (he and she, him and her).
9. Neither the child nor the parents want (his, their) files reviewed.
10. The doctor, along with his assistants, will operate on (his, their) patient.

EXERCISE 5-6: Complete each sentence to include a pronoun that refers to an antecedent. Proofread to ensure the pronoun agrees with its antecedent.

1. Neither the __________ nor the ______________________________
____.
2. How do the ______________________________________?
3. Each patient ______________________________________.
4. The clinic ______________________________________.
5. Two patients ______________________________________.

DANGLING MODIFIERS

A dangling modifier is a group of words that is misplaced because this group does not modify the intended word. These often occur at the beginning of the sentence; however, a dangling modifier can occur elsewhere in the sentence. For example,

Singing in the tree, the long-term care <u>resident</u> watched the bird.

The sentence should read:

The long-term care <u>resident</u> watched the bird singing in the tree.

We understand the bird was in the tree, not the resident.

EXERCISE 5-7: Read the sentences and place a check in front of those sentences that have a dangling modifier.

________ 1. Having completed the assignment, the list was reviewed by the certified nursing assistant.

________ 2. Calling the patient's family, the nurse was delighted with the patient's condition.

________ 3. The bandage by pouring warm water over the incision site was removed by the nurse.

________ 4. After completing multiple tests, the report was sent to the doctor by the laboratory assistant.

________ 5. Lacking O positive blood, the patient's surgery was delayed.

EXERCISE 5-8: Revise the sentences to remove the dangling modifiers.

1. After reading the article about Paxil, the information was helpful to the patient.

____

____

2. The chart, recovering from the procedure, is placed at the foot of the patient's bed.

___

___

3. Hanging the IV, the pole needed to be stabilized by the nurse.

___

___

4. The medical receptionist compiled a letter, drafting the complaint to the insurance company.

___

___

5. The diagnosis refusing to believe the doctor upset the family.

___

___

6. Eating the balanced diet, the nutritious foods took on a new meaning for the young diabetics.

___

___

7. Twisting the patient in a variety of positions, the muscles were viewed in a variety of positions by the physical therapists.

___

___

8. Scanning the lumbar region, the MRI was used by the technician to locate the growth.

___

___

9. Flossing daily, the teeth and gums are cleaned below the gum line.

___

___

10. Massaging the swollen area, the pain slowly dissipated.

___

___

PARALLEL STRUCTURE

To have parallel structure in a sentence means to have equality and coordination between words and groups of words. Writers pair equal grammatical units to make a sentence parallel. To achieve parallel structure, a writer matches noun and noun, verb and verb, prepositional phrase and prepositional phrase. In the case of parallel structure and verbs, the verbs must be in the same tense. For example,

The dietitian oversees the dietary helpers and creates the diet plans. (present-tense verb + adjective + noun)

The patient, forlorn and tearful, wanted to return home. (adjective + adjective)

The pharmacy technician and medical assistant studied anatomy and physiology. (noun + noun)

So, writers use their knowledge of grammar to ensure that similar ideas are reflected by the similar grammatical structures in sentences.

EXERCISE 5-9: Underline the parallel structures in these sentences.

1. The patient has the right to know his prognosis and the need to know the medical implications.
2. In the morning and in the afternoon, the shift reports are conducted in Room 125.
3. The refusal to take the medicine and the desire to return home were her most common subjects of discussion.
4. The patient is stable and mobile.
5. The rehabilitation assistant ambulated the patient and then massaged the patient's legs after the walk this morning.
6. Removing the gauze and cleaning the wound, the nurse described the steps and showed the patient the method of wound care.
7. Changing colostomy bags takes skill and requires patience with new patients.
8. When the patient is angry and frustrated, the caregiver reminds the patient of his need to be motivated.
9. Human emotions and human behavior tell a great deal about the health of a patient.
10. Common sense and problem-solving logic can help a young mother determine when to call the doctor and when to wait before calling the doctor.

EXERCISE 5-10: Correct the errors in parallel structure in these sentences.

1. He wants to have peace of mind and avoidance of stress.

____

____

2. The nurse wanted to speak with the parents and told them about the therapy session.

3. The physician's assistant was tired, cold, and wanted to eat something.

4. The supervisor tried to be helpful, encouraged and supporting of his team.

5. In an exhaustive search and reading lots of medical journals, the information about the procedure was found.

6. The lack of personal care and of resources left the patient in poor condition before the surgery.

7. The doctor told the patient to schedule a follow-up appointment, but the patient decides that another visit is not necessary.

8. The patient was uncomfortable and dissatisfaction with the care he was given.

9. The treatments options were discussed with the patient and her family; the decision is made a week ago to begin chemotherapy.

10. The clerical staff type, copy, file, and then need to mail their daily work.

VERB TENSE

The most common verb tenses seen in medical journals, textbooks, and common usage are the simple present tense, the simple past tense, and the present perfect tense. Each has its own form and usage rules. Verb tense places an action as a fact or general truth or an action in time. Writers tend to use the present tense the most. Present tense is used to present research, information, and facts for journal articles and textbooks because the present tense is ageless; whenever the passage is read, the information is presented as fact or habit.

Typically, present tense is used in articles to provide information. For example,

Two million cases of leishmania occur around the world each year.

The tumor is malignant.

If a specific event occurred in the past, then the past tense is used. The past tense sets the event in a previous time. For example,

Uncle Bill had a stroke in 1988.

The surgeon completed the procedure at 4:00 P.M.

If the action started in the past and continues into the present time, use the present perfect. This tense shows duration more than a specific time. For example,

We have provided constant care for our mother.

The research on stem cells has continued despite the unknowns.

Being consistent in using verb tense is important. When a writer changes tense in a sentence, it can confuse the reader. For example,

The doctor goes to his office, and he worked there until noon.

This sentence is strange because as a reader we understand that both verbs should be in the past tense. This sentence relays information about a previous event and not a habit. Thus it should read:

The doctor went to his office, and he worked there until noon.

However, the following sentence does show habitual or usual activity:

Dr. Brown arrives at the hospital at 9:00 each day.

Below is a summary of the uses and forms of verbs.

Tense	Graphic	When to Use It/Form	Examples
Present (base form of verb)		A habit or usual activity A general truth A scientific fact Summarizing an article	He lives a simple life. Diet is important to health. The child brushes his teeth twice a day.
Past (verb + *ed* or irregular ending)		An event that started and ended at a specific time in the past	The device performed met with his new receptionist this morning.

Future (<u>*will*</u> + present verb tense form)		An event that will start and end at a specific time in the future	The rehabilitation therapist <u>will meet</u> with the family at 2 o'clock today.
Present Perfect (*has/have* + past participle of the verb)		An event starts in the past and continues into the present	The patient <u>has recovered</u> nicely. We <u>have learned</u> to work together as a medical team.

EXERCISE 5-11: Read the following sentences. If a shift in tense or an incorrect use of tense occurs, place an *X* on the blank by the sentence.

_______ **1.** The physician saw patients between 7:00 A.M. and 9:30 A.M. six days a week.

_______ **2.** When I need to see the dentist, I went to the closest one to my home.

_______ **3.** The patient was already prepared for the procedure; it will begin in about three minutes.

_______ **4.** The surgery proceeded as planned and scheduled.

_______ **5.** Our office closes next April for a remodeling project.

EXERCISE 5-12: Use each term in a present-tense sentence.

1. bathe ______________________________

2. suture ______________________________

3. massage ______________________________

4. bandage ______________________________

5. test ______________________________

EXERCISE 5-13: Use each term in a past-tense sentence.

1. examine ______________________________

2. remove ______________________________

3. swipe ______________________________

4. excise ______________________________

5. trim ______________________________

Exercise 5-14: Use each term in a present-perfect sentence.

1. input ______________________________

2. inspire ______________________________

3. make ______________________________

4. eat ______________________________

5. clip ______________________________

UNIT PROOFREADING EXERCISES

Read the following paragraph and correct any errors in subject–verb agreement, pronoun–antecedent agreement, verb tense, dangling modifiers, parallel structure, and grammar.

Burns have been classified as first, second, or third degree depending on its depth not how much pain or damage has been done. A first-degree burn reached the outer layer of skin. In this case, the skin appear dry, painful, and sensitive to touch a sunburn was an example of a first-degree burn. A second-degree burn has damaged several layers of skin. The skin may became swoll, puffy, weeping, or blistered. One example of a second-degree burn might be a hot-water burn. A third-degree burn, involved all layers of the skin and any underlying tissue and/or organs, has resulted in dry, pale white or charred black, swollen skin. Damaging or destroying the nerve, the patient may experience no or little pain. Third-degree burns need immediate medical attention.

UNIT REVISION EXERCISES

Each sentence below has one error in verb or pronoun usage or structure. Locate each error and revise the sentence.

1. Every one of the patients in this section of the wing need to receive his medication.
2. Either of the drugs are used to treat this condition.

3. Not only is the doctor working in the hospital but in the residential community clinic too.
4. The patient needs to be bathed and attending the physical therapy session scheduled for 9:30 A.M.
5. Microbiology was the scientific study of microorganisms.

UNIT EXTENSIONS

1. Read this long legal declaration for mental health treatment. Then rewrite it in common language and short sentences that are parallel in structure.

   I, _______________, being an adult of sound mind, willfully and voluntarily make this request for mental health treatment to be followed if it is determined by a court of law that my ability to understand the nature and consequences of a proposed treatment, including the benefits, risks, and alternatives to the proposed treatment, is impaired to such an extent that I lack the capacity to make mental health treatment decisions.

2. Look at the patient health form provided below and then draft five sentences that provide the patient's complaints and the symptoms associated with each complaint.

Meadow Villa Clinic	
Michael Smith	Age 54 Gender [X] Male [ ] Female
19875 South 4th Avenue	Phone: 202-555-0100
Portland, Oregon	Insurance: South Sound HMO
Allergies: none	Group/ID #: C234-987550
Medications: none Have you recently had: Headaches [X] Yes [ ] No Increased work stress [X] Yes [ ] No Change in lifestyle [X] Yes [ ] No Anxiety [X] Yes [ ] No	Chief Complaint: I have been unable to sleep. My eyes run and my nose is stuffed up. I am very nervous and can't relax. People bother me a lot. I have stomachaches, and I eat all the time. I am worried about my job. I might lose it. I feel tired all the time. My concentration is gone. The other day I could not remember my phone

(continued)

Depression	☒ Yes ☐ No	number. I was so upset because my ex-wife called to say that I had missed my pickup time of the kids. I feel so tired and upset. I have been getting hives and just being out of sorts.
Weight Loss	☒ Yes ☐ No	
Weight Gain	☐ Yes ☒ No	

3. Medical offices are going to digitalization. Sometimes digital patient records may be required by new regulatory compliance rules such as insurance coverage and documentation. About 85% of hospitals in the United States are still using paper-based systems despite the availability of reliable information technology. A paperless system would allow for more efficient processing of patient records and insurance claims. A paperless system would improve the speed, access, and accuracy of handling records daily. Go to the Internet and learn about this issue, then take a stance pro or con. Defend your point with facts.

UNIT 5 SELF-CHECK

1. Explain what a dangling modifier is. Why is a dangling modifier an error in sentence structure?

____

____

____

Read the sentences below. If the sentence is correct, mark *C* on the line. If it is incorrect, mark *W* on the line, then make the corrections in the sentence.

_______ **2.** Each of the phlebotomists complete 100 blood draws this morning.

_______ **3.** The cryoprobe is a device that apply cold to tissue.

_______ **4.** Eating a diet rich in fruits and vegetables are healthy and nutritious.

_______ **5.** Sixty pounds are a lot of weight to lose.

_______ **6.** That safety harness is too loose.

_______ **7.** Surgical instruments and equipment must be properly sterilized.

_______ **8.** Infusion are one of the methods of dispensing medications.

_______ **9.** Pediatric patients need to feel secure, loved, and being nurtured.

_______ **10.** One of the keloids are growing rapidly.

_______ **11.** Economics are involved in our decision to keep our insurance provider.

_______ **12.** The doctor, along with his staff members, report to the hospital board.

UNIT 6

Achieving More in Sentence Variety

UNIT TERMS

Appositive phrase	A group of words that describes the noun that precedes it; usually consists of adjectives and nouns
Base verb	The simple present tense of the verb
Gerunds	Verbal phrases that use a verb to form a noun construction (base verb + *-ing*)
Infinitives	Verbal phrases that use a verb to form a noun, adjective, or adverb construction (*to* + verb)
Participles	Verbal phrases that use a verb to form an adjective construction (verb + *-ed*, *-en*, or *-ing*)

UNIT OBJECTIVES

Upon completion of this unit, the student will be able to

1. identify a gerund, infinitive, participial phrase in a sentence
2. write a sentence that includes a gerund
3. write a sentence that includes an infinitive
4. write a sentence that includes a participial phrase
5. revise sentences to reflect the conceptual thinking of the writer
6. incorporate appositive phrases to shorten adjective clauses

Glossary of Medical Terms

Term	Part of Speech	Definition
alleviate	verb	to get rid of; to relieve; to improve
allied health	noun	a healthcare worker who is part of a healthcare team
caplet	noun	a small oval tablet
dental hygienist	noun	a licensed specialist trained in the prevention of dental disease and in the cleaning and health of teeth
deterioration	noun	a decline in health or condition
drape	verb; noun	to cover; a covering for privacy or warmth
health–illness continuum	noun	the measure of health; the presence or absence of health or well-being

meditate	verb	to think deeply, to concentrate
MRI	noun	magnetic resonance imaging; a type of diagnostic radiography
mononucleosis	noun	an illness caused by an abnormally high number of mononuclear leukocytes (white blood cells) in the blood
ophthalmic assistant	noun	one who assists the ophthalmologist
pediatrician	noun	a specialist in children's diseases
pharmacy technician	noun	one who assists the pharmacist
radiologist	noun	a physician who specializes in X-rays and other radiation sources for diagnosis and treatment of disease
sputum	noun	a substance produced by coughing or clearing one's throat
swollen	adjective	enlarged or distended
urologist	noun	a physician specializing in the urinary tract

Changing sentences from weak constructions to strong constructions takes a little practice and consideration of the sentence structure. The first addition to sentences to vary their structure is to incorporate the verbal phrases of gerunds, infinitives, and participials. These phrases serve to expand basic sentence structure by allowing the writer to communicate ideas in a sophisticated manner.

GERUNDS

To Form a Gerund	Function	Example
Base verb + *-ing*	Use it as a noun that indicates an activity.	Dieting requires self-control.

Gerunds are always nouns. Like nouns, a gerund may function as the subject of a sentence, direct object, or the object of a preposition:

Dieting requires self-control. (subject—provides the actor of the sentence)

She started dieting. (direct object—completes the verb's action)

He lost thirteen pounds by dieting. (object of the preposition)

Gerunds are a way to vary sentence structure without a lot of effort. This structure is solid and straightforward to achieve. Usually a gerund at the start of a sentence helps direct the reader's attention to a specific activity or topic.

EXERCISE 6-1: Underline each gerund in the following sentences.

1. Talking to his visitors is how the patient spent his afternoon.
2. The radiologist appears to be reviewing the X-rays.
3. The residents of the long-term care facility enjoy talking with their doctors.

4. Working in a medical office is her preference.
5. By studying medical terminology, the clerks are more efficient in reviewing medical reports and documents.

EXERCISE 6-2: Complete these sentences that have gerunds in them.

1. Wiping the edges of the wound requires ______________________________

____

2. By seeing the film, the allied health students were ________________

____

3. Giving a patient a bed bath helps ______________________________

____

4. By not eating, the patient had ________________________________

____

5. Transferring patients takes __________________________________

____

EXERCISE 6-3: Draft sentences with the following verbs as gerunds and use these gerunds in the specified format.

1. diagnose

____

____

2. massage

____

____

3. refer

____

____

4. prescribe

____

____

5. input

____

____

Exercise 6-4: Revise the sentences below to include a gerund. You may need to rephrase parts of the sentences; however, attempt to maintain a similar meaning.

1. The promotion of a patient's independence is critical in assisting him to meet his healthcare needs.

   ____

   ____

2. It is important to try to understand a patient's cultural background, for it allows healthcare professionals to understand the person's behavior.

   ____

   ____

3. The plan for job duties and responsibilities for the new position should alleviate stress among the staff.

   ____

   ____

4. It is important to identify alternatives for treatments for all patients, and it is part of his job.

   ____

   ____

5. The direction of information is the job of the center's administrator.

   ____

   ____

6. In order to avoid legal suits, nursing staff should be knowledgeable of the patient's rights.

   ____

   ____

7. To care for the elderly takes a special person.

   ____

   ____

8. We hope to locate her closest relative, which may be difficult.

   ____

   ____

9. We expanded our diagnostic procedures to cover the national guidelines.

   ____

   ____

10. To wash one's hands is important to prevent the transfer of bacteria.

   ____

   ____

INFINITIVES

To Form an Infinitive	Function	Example
To + base verb	Use it as a noun, adjective, or adverb.	To diet takes patience. The doctor to see is Dr. Sheila Houser. The patient ambulated to regain his balance.

An infinitive begins with the word *to* and is followed by the simple form of a verb. Some examples are *to eat, to assist the patient, to inform the doctor, to practice balancing*. Each example includes *to* plus a simple verb. Additional words may contribute to a phrase as in *to prepare the medicine cart* or *to assist the patient in relearning certain skills*. A common error occurs when an infinitive phrase is confused with a prepositional phrase beginning with the word *to*. Remember that a prepositional phrase includes a preposition and a noun, as in *to the store, to the waiting area, to central supply*. Verbs are never part of prepositional phrases. Infinitives can function as nouns, adjectives, or adverbs:

To swallow a caplet is easier than you think. (subject)

The medicine to be prescribed is a sedative. (adjective describing medicine)

The doctor prescribed a diet to help control her eating habits. (adverb explaining under what condition the person is prescribed a diet)

Most common for healthcare applications will be the infinitive used as a subject or as an adjective.

EXERCISE 6-5: Underline each infinitive in the following sentences.

1. To review the screenings is her job.
2. The doctor to see is your primary care physician.
3. He wants to speak with his urologist sometime today.
4. The reason to be concerned is the rapid deterioration of the skin.
5. The doctor will call to schedule the lab work.

EXERCISE 6-6: Label the infinitive by function: noun, adjective, or adverb.

1. ________ The tooth to be filled is a molar.
2. ________ To schedule the appointment, call the office after 8:00 A.M.
3. ________ The MRI to be taken is scheduled for Monday at 9:00 A.M.
4. ________ The doctor asked the patient to call his office in two days.
5. ________ The nurses saved their money to have a party for the interns.

6. _______ <u>To be allowed to go home early</u> required the patient's family to be available to assist him.

7. _______ We wish <u>to travel as VISTA nurses.</u>

8. _______ Our collaborative efforts <u>to give support</u> aided in the patient's recovery.

9. _______ We advised him <u>to seek treatment as soon as possible</u>.

10. _______ <u>To have empathy</u> is a workplace skill.

EXERCISE 6-7: Complete these sentences that have infinitives in them.

1. To relieve muscle tension _______________________________
2. To inform your supervisor _______________________________
3. _______________________________ to improve his position.
4. _______________ to study _______________
5. The reason to be concerned is _______________________________

EXERCISE 6-8: Draft sentences using the following verbs as infinitives in the specified format.

1. diagnose

____

____

2. transport

____

____

3. divide

____

____

4. cure

____

____

5. inject

____

____

EXERCISE 6-9: Revise the sentences below to include an infinitive. You may need to rephrase parts of the sentences; however, attempt to maintain a similar meaning.

1. The two clavicles help by bracing the shoulders and prevent forward motion.

2. The medical assistant kept busy by calling patients reminding them of their upcoming appointments.

3. Lifting properly prevents back injuries.

4. The nurse will be reviewing the patient care plan as part of her duties.

5. The dentist is thinking about requesting the dental assistants be available for attending an after-work meeting.

6. Warming up is important before exercising vigorously.

7. Requesting that patients complete the health survey is part of our quality-assurance plan.

8. Discussing confidential information in the staff room is strictly against policy.

9. Writing thank-you notes to the community volunteers is important.

10. Having your name removed from our mailing list is a quick procedure.

PARTICIPLES

To Form a Participial Phrase	Function	Example
Base verb + *–ed*	Use it as an adjective.	The patient, bothered by the noise, complained.
Base verb + *–en*		Broken at the joint, the finger has swollen.
Base verb + *–ing*		Giggling with her mom, the child was feeling better.

Participles are two main parts of the verb. The present participle is the verb plus *–ing*, as in *I am* ______+ *–ing*, as in *I am seeing the doctor*. The past participle is the verb plus *–ed*, *–en*, or *–t*, as in *I have looked* and *I have slept*. These examples are verbs; however, as a verbal, the participle must function as an adjective:

The nurse is scheduling appointments. (verb)

Scheduling the appointment, the nurse assisted the patient. (adjective)

Participial phrases always begin with the participle and then end in modifiers or objects. They are often set off by commas and are followed or preceded by the noun the participle is modifying:

Working four ten-hour shifts, the healthcare worker felt happy to have three days off each week.

The healthcare provider, using three different billing systems, was anxious to purchase a uniform system to be used throughout all of its facilities.

A common error occurs if the participle is not immediately followed or preceded by the noun it is modifying. When the noun does not follow or precede the participle, this error is called a dangling modifier:

Waiting for the appointment spreadsheet, the computer shut down on the medical receptionist. (Incorrect)

Rewrite to correct the error:

Waiting for the appointment spreadsheet, the medical receptionist noticed that her computer shut down.

EXERCISE 6-10: Identify the participial phrases in the sentences.

1. Working as a medical assistant, she is content.
2. The patient, having lived alone for years, is having a difficult time adjusting to the group home.
3. Handing out the magazines, the volunteers provide a friendly face for the patients.

4. The wheelchair, broken and without a battery, needs to go to the repair center.

5. Removing his contacts, the patient is ready for the eyedrops.

EXERCISE 6-11: Complete these sentences that contain participial phrases.

1. Hugging her mother in the recovery room, ______________________________

____

2. Removing the gauze, ____

____

3. Rubbing the patient's back, ____

____

4. The nurse, asking the visitors to wait outside the room, ______________

____

5. Covering the patient with a drape, ____________________________________

____

6. The doctor, speaking in a quiet voice, _________________________________

____

7. The dental hygienist, wanting to ensure a proper exam, ______________

____

8. The ophthalmic assistant, handing the wand to the patient, ____________

____

9. ____

wanting the patient to recover quickly ______________________________

10. The allied health instructor, repeating the critical information, __________

____

EXERCISE 6-12: Draft sentences with the following verbs as participles in the specified format.

1. diagnose

____

____

2. transport

____

____

3. divide

4. cure

5. inject

Another way to use participles is to rewrite an adjective clause as a participial. Ensure that the participial is placed next to the noun or pronoun that it modifies:

The student *who is studying to be a pharmacy technician* is also interested in nursing.

Studying to be a pharmacy technician, the student is also interested in nursing.

Exercise 6-13: Revise the sentences below to include a participle. You may need to rephrase parts of the sentences; however, attempt to maintain a similar meaning.

1. The patient, who refused to believe the test results, sought a second opinion.

2. The student was unable to remember the car accident; he led police to believe that he wasn't driving.

3. The family members will learn to cope with his death, and they continue their pursuit of cancer research.

4. A nurse should possess the ability to educate the patient for self-care and health maintenance.

5. It is important for a patient to understand the health–illness continuum because it shows that there is no specific point of wellness or illness.

6. Pediatricians encourage mothers to teach their children the importance of wearing seat belts, for it saves lives.

7. The eye-care profession hopes to create optimal vision for the patients. The sophisticated measurement devices are used.

8. Eyeglass prescriptions always have a spherical power. These powers are calculated by a technician to the patient's specifications.

9. The woman is on a diet. She hopes to reduce her body fat by 5%. She walks for exercise each day.

10. Youths drink too much soda and sugared beverages. They are missing essential nutrients and the benefits of water.

The key to differentiating gerunds and participles is understanding their function and location. Observe where each of these occurs in the sentence and their corresponding punctuation. Gerunds typically aren't separated off from the sentence by commas as participial phrases are. Participles provide extra information because they are adjectives. If you cross out the verb + *-ing* phrase and the sentence is still complete, then the phrase is a participial phrase. Gerunds are nouns and therefore, unless used as the noun in a prepositional phrase, are a required part of a sentence.

IMPROVING STYLE

Weak sentences include a variety of constructions that need to be modified. Exact wording will express your specific point. Avoid vague terms and constructions. Use positive terms to frame content, rather than negative terms:

It is the patient's request to seek a second opinion.

The patient requests a second opinion.

The thing that bothers her most is her mother's aphasia.

Her mother's aphasia bothers her most.

One strategy to assist you in writing more specific sentences is to use medical terms and specific phrases used in the healthcare field.

To improve the precision of your writing, follow these steps:

1. Remove and revise the beginning of sentences to avoid *it* and *there* as sentence starters:

   It is advised that the patient should not participate in vigorous activity.

   The patient should not participate in vigorous activity.

2. Remove unnecessary words expressing quantity:

   The incision site contains a total of sixteen staples.

   The incision site contains sixteen staples.

3. Replace weak verbs with strong, specific ones. Weak verbs include *do, make, get*, and forms of *be*. Use the verb that expresses the specific activity:

   This textbook section is an explanation of how to adjust IV drips.

   This textbook section explains how to adjust IV drips.

4. Replace expressions that serve no purpose in communicating the basic message:

   Align the patient's body in such a manner that his spine is straight.

   Align the patient's body so his spine is straight.

5. Replace negative words with positive ones. Try to ensure a "can-do" attitude in the choice of words and phrases used:

   I <u>don't have much</u> work experience.

   My work experience is limited, but I am eager to learn.

EXERCISE 6-14: Revise these sentences to ensure more specific expression and to ensure a positive "can-do" tone.

1. For this procedure, there are eight steps that must be carried out.

   ____

   ____

2. It is assumed that this individual is a hypochondriac.

   ____

   ____

3. There is a dental assistant who tells everybody how important brushing and flossing are to do.

   ____

   ____

4. He wants to try the task even if it is difficult.

____

____

5. My coworkers are lazy when the boss isn't around.

____

____

6. Some patients are so picky.

____

____

7. That sputum stinks.

____

____

8. He has to pee a lot.

____

____

9. I hate to lift heavy items.

____

____

10. That is not my job.

____

____

UNIT PROOFREADING EXERCISES

Read the following passage and make corrections for errors in punctuation, spelling, syntax, exact language, and other sentence errors.

Mononucleosis is referred to as "mono" or the "kissing disease." And is a viral infection. It is common in older teenagers and young adults. I believe it is most commonly characterized by a sore sore throat and fatigue. Other sympotoms include weakness dizziness swollen lymph glans and an in larged spleen. It is diagnosed by a blood test. This disease may last several weeks or so. There is no specific treat ment accept rest plenty of fluids and aspiring for body aches. If infected, glasses and silverware should not be shared.

UNIT REVISION EXERCISES

Revise these sentences to improve their content and style.

1. The man, who is a dermatologist, encourages his patients to drink at least 64 ounces of water each day.

2. There is not a single reason for his unexplainable illness.

3. The man wanted to capture each moment with his grandchildren, so he videotaped them each time they visited him in the hospital.

4. It is important that we exercise daily and avoid too many junk foods.

5. I believe that my struggle with trying to quit smoking has affected my lifestyle.

UNIT EXTENSIONS

1. Do an Internet search for information on crack-addicted babies. Develop a PowerPoint slide show providing statistics, signs, and social policy dealing with this healthcare issue.
2. Look inside your food pantry. Locate the ingredients needed to make a main dish. Calculate the entire meal's nutritional values and calories. Note its nutritional strengths and weaknesses. Make suggestions for improving the nutritional content.
3. Pretend that you are a professional advice giver like Dear Abby. Respond to a letter from a healthcare student who writes to you complaining that there are too many facts, details, and specifics to memorize in the healthcare field.

UNIT 6 SELF-CHECK

Identify the phrase in each sentence. Underline and label each phrase. Use the following labels: appositive phrase *(AP)*, gerund phrase *(GP)*, infinitive phrase *(IP)*, participial phrase *(PaP)*, prepositional phrase *(PP)*, and verb phrase *(VP)*.

Patient Bob was admitted to the emergency room. Complaining of stomach pains, the patient explained that at first he thought he had overeaten. To his dismay, the pains became more and more severe. He felt that he needed to call his doctor. The doctor's answering service recommended that he go to the emergency room. The attending physician, an internal medicine specialist, felt that he was having a bout with diverticulitis. The doctor ordered several tests, run by the hospital lab, to determine the cause of his pain. Soon a round of antibiotics was ordered, and Bob was allowed to go home. Being released from the emergency room, Bob was feeling better.

UNIT 7

Paragraph Basics

UNIT TERMS

Concluding sentence	A sentence that helps draw the paragraph to a close
Indentation	One tab or about five single spaces at the beginning of a paragraph
Support sentence	Sentences that support the topic sentence
Topic sentence	Also called the main-idea sentence; provides the central idea and direction to the paragraph
Transition word	A word or group of words that helps join ideas or sentences

UNIT OBJECTIVES

Upon completion of this unit, the student will be able to

1. recognize the parts of a paragraph
2. draft a topic sentence that is effective
3. draft paragraphs using text question prompts
4. revise and improve paragraphs

Glossary of Medical Terms

Term	Part of Speech	Definition
anus	noun	the outlet of the rectum, the outer opening of the intestines
appetite	noun	a desire for food or to eat
chronic	adjective	of long duration
communicable disease	noun	a disease transmitted from one person to another
digestive tract	noun	the tract from the mouth to the anus
exploratory	adjective	examination of a body part or organ
noninvasive	adjective	not likely to spread; or can describe a device, examination, or procedure that doesn't enter the body
obesity	noun	abnormal amount of body fat
pinworms	noun	parasitic worms that live in the intestine and rectum
rectum	noun	the lower end of the intestine
remedy	noun	a cure for a disease or something to relieve it
ultrasound	noun	inaudible sound used in diagnostic procedures to outline the shape of an organ or tissue
ultrasonography	noun	use of ultrasound to produce an image or photograph of an organ or tissue

PARTS OF A PARAGRAPH

As writers, we use paragraphs in so many different ways. Paragraphs can help us communicate in a brief note, a short letter, a memo, and for course work. All paragraphs have parts that help the reader understand the main idea and its support.

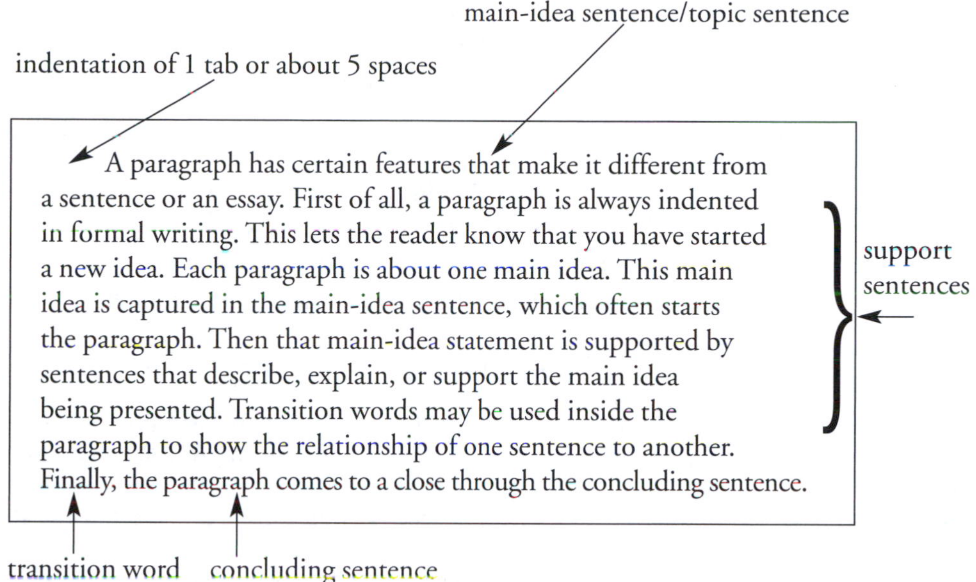

main-idea sentence/topic sentence
indentation of 1 tab or about 5 spaces
A paragraph has certain features that make it different from a sentence or an essay. First of all, a paragraph is always indented in formal writing. This lets the reader know that you have started a new idea. Each paragraph is about one main idea. This main idea is captured in the main-idea sentence, which often starts the paragraph. Then that main-idea statement is supported by sentences that describe, explain, or support the main idea being presented. Transition words may be used inside the paragraph to show the relationship of one sentence to another. Finally, the paragraph comes to a close through the concluding sentence.
support sentences
transition word
concluding sentence

A paragraph is a set of sentences that pertain to one subject or topic. A paragraph has three distinct parts: a topic or main-idea sentence, supporting sentences, and a concluding sentence. Each paragraph should be indented approximately five spaces or one tab of five spaces.

A topic sentence or main-idea sentence expresses the main point of the paragraph and provides the controlling idea of the paragraph's content. In addition, the topic sentence can show your breadth of knowledge of a term, condition, procedure, or situation. The words and phrases direct the reader's attention to the level of detail and direction of thought. So, the focus and word choice are important. The supporting sentences provide the reasons that support your main-idea sentence. These reasons are further illustrated with examples, details, anecdotes, and explanations. Supporting sentences illustrate and prove the point of your main-idea sentence.

The concluding sentence brings the thought on that specific topic to a close; it may recap or emphasize the main point in a variety of ways. For example, it may provide the reader with a summary of the main idea, or it can leave the reader with something to think about: How will this impact me? What did I learn? What does this mean? Generally speaking, the concluding sentence does not include any new information on the topic, although it may serve as a tie to the next paragraph.

EXERCISE 7-1: Label the parts of the paragraph below. Use the following labels: topic sentence, support sentences, concluding sentence.

The development of ultrasonography has played a major role in noninvasive test procedures for diagnostic purposes. Ultrasonography is a technique that reflects high-frequency sound waves off internal tissues. A transducer, a detection device, locates and converts ultrasonic waves into electrical impulses. These impulses are then displayed on a video monitor and can be recorded for future evaluation. Ultrasonography is easy, inexpensive, and quick to administer. Little or no risk is presented to the patient. With this diagnostic technique, we are able to see internal tissue images, although not always clearly, without having to conduct time-consuming and expensive exploratory surgery. Patients and healthcare professionals alike benefit from this innovation.

Drafting topic sentences can take some practice. First of all, it is important to understand that the topic sentence states the main idea for the entire paragraph. The topic sentence controls the content of the entire paragraph. Two important parts should be provided in a topic sentence:

1. a narrowed subject on a specific topic or responding to a specific question
2. a controlling idea that helps control the information included in the paragraph. This is the central point that you are making about the subject.

The following is an example of a weak topic sentence:

Nurses need to be detail oriented.

This topic is neither narrow nor controlling. The reader has no idea what information will be included in the paragraph. Below is a revised topic sentence:

Nurses play a critical role in ensuring patient care; therefore, the nurse must be detail oriented in the care provided, in the instructions given to the patient, and in documentation of the care given.

Use the following guidelines as a measure of topic sentence effectiveness:

1. The topic sentence includes a controlling idea.
2. The topic sentence controls the paragraph's content.
3. The topic sentence reflects an accurate message either in response to a prompt or question or provides your point clearly.

Exercise 7-2: Review these topic sentences. Mark whether each is effective or ineffective.

1. Healthcare is an important subject. ☐ effective ☐ ineffective
2. Without a solid patient–client relationship, the healthcare provider may be limited in understanding the patient's needs. ☐ effective ☐ ineffective
3. I really want to be a medical assistant. ☐ effective ☐ ineffective
4. More research into the links among diet, exercise, and genetics will provide answers to a means of slowing the onset of chronic heart disease. ☐ effective ☐ ineffective

5. I think that the healthcare industry is booming. ☐ effective ☐ ineffective
6. Most people do not know that secondhand smoke kills 38,000 American each year. ☐ effective ☐ ineffective
7. Drug-addicted babies have a right to a safe home environment and excellent medical care. ☐ effective ☐ ineffective
8. Communicable diseases aren't common today. ☐ effective ☐ ineffective
9. A trip to the magazine aisle helped me realize that healthcare offers vast career choices. ☐ effective ☐ ineffective
10. Germs are bad. ☐ effective ☐ ineffective

EXERCISE 7-3: Write a topic sentence of your own for each topic below. Use the guidelines to assist your writing.

1. Introduce yourself by featuring one of your unique features or characteristics.
2. Explain why you have chosen a career in the health professions.
3. What does "quality of life" mean to you?
4. Explain your interpretation of the saying, "You are only as old as you feel."
5. How will your personal character strengths benefit the profession you have chosen?

EXERCISE 7-4: Develop one of the above topic sentences into a paragraph.

____
____
____
____
____
____
____
____
____
____
____
____
____
____
____

Once your paragraph is written, use the list below to assist you in ensuring that you have created an effective paragraph. The paragraph must:

- ☐ be on topic
- ☐ be indented
- ☐ be legible
- ☐ have a topic or main-idea sentence
- ☐ have adequate support sentences with examples, details, and rationale
- ☐ have a concluding sentence
- ☐ be written in a mature manner with sophisticated and varied sentence structures

TEST TAKING AND THE PARAGRAPH

Writing for classroom assignments and tests requires one to be specific and organized. The information that is given must be easily understood, logical, and accurate.

Oftentimes, a context provided by a paragraph helps make the answer easier to read and comprehend. In such situations, follow these basic guidelines:

1. *Read the question carefully.* Underline the key words and phrases that tell you what is being asked. As you write your answer, refer back to these words and phrases to ensure that you are still on topic and answering the question.

   Become familiar with the key words of test questions:

Term	As a writer, you should:
Analyze	Divide the subject into parts and show their relationships. Explain how the parts work individually and as a whole.
Compare	Search for the similarities. Examine the individual characteristics to determine the similarities.
Contrast	Search for the differences. Examine the individual characteristics to determine the differences.
Define	Provide a meaning. Avoid generalization. Use specific features to distinguish the term from all others.
Enumerate	Provide a list of items. Order the list appropriately to reflect the importance or sequence of activities.
Evaluate	Judge the positive and negative aspects of something. Avoid emotional language or biases. Be clinical. Rely on known procedures and policies to ensure validity.
Explain	Provide details and make the topic understandable. Use clear instructions. Avoid assuming that your reader knows. Get to the point.

Identify	Provide the characteristics or features of something and its importance. Be clinical and avoid emotive language.
Interpret	Explain the meaning of something. Show the relationship among the parts. Rely on data and facts to support the explanation.

2. *Get organized.* Jot down a few ideas and focus on what your answer to the question will be. By drafting a list, you will include the specific details to support the answer.
3. *Give specific examples and supporting evidence for the test question.* Tailor your choice of examples to fit the question. Your general statements must be supported with clear and concise examples, specific details, and succinct rationale and evidence.
4. *Answer in paragraph format.* Indent five spaces and make the paragraph easy to read. The paragraph format will help you avoid adding random details or straying from the topic. Furthermore, it will provide a context for the answer.

What should a paragraph for a test question look like?

The first sentence of the paragraph should be the basic answer to the question. You may have a lot to say about the topic; however, this sentence should direct and control the answer of the question. This one sentence should tell the reader that you know the answer. Then move into the reasons for this answer by providing details, rationale, and other evidence. These may be medical facts, theories that support the answer, or drug interaction information from a text. The supporting sentences should provide the details and examples that support the very first sentence. A standard paragraph has between three and six supporting sentences. The final sentence is the concluding sentence, which brings the paragraph to a close. No new information is added in the conclusion; instead, the information already provided may be reflected on, summarized, or connected to other information that you have studied as long as it is relevant.

Exercise 7-5: Write a test-question response in paragraph form. Choose one and respond.

1. What are three specific reasons for obesity in America?
2. What is the largest threat to the public health of Americans?
3. Why are there so many people not covered by insurance in this country?
4. Do grocery stores hold some responsibility for the food choices people make?

____

____

____

____

____

____

____

____

____

____

____

____

____

____

____

____

____

____

____

____

____

____

____

____

____

____

____

____

____

____

____

____

UNIT PROOFREADING EXERCISES

Read the following paragraph. Correct any errors in the grammar, punctuation, and paragraph format.

Pinworms are tiny thread like worms. They infect the digestive tract of young children. Common among 4- to 6-year-old children, but anyone can become infected. Pinworms live in the upper portion of the intestine and they travel outside the anus to lay their eggs. Which occurs at night and causes the child to itch. These eggs are able to live outside the body for days on clothing and bedding and this is how other family members can become infected. If a child scratches the rectum area and then sucks his thumb; reinfection occurs. If a parent suspects an infection, he should enter the bedroom at night and shine a flashlight on the child anus. The light will make the worms move back to the anus. Over the counter remedies exist. Wash bedding and sleeping clothes. Encourage hand washing and keep fingernails short. In a severe case, the child may complain about stomach pains and experience a lost of appetite.

UNIT REVISION EXERCISES

This paragraph is in response to a test question on a first-quarter exam. You may edit and revise the paragraph in any way that improves it to meet the guidelines for effective paragraph writing. Write the revision on lined paper.

Assignment: Select one medical diagnostic technique and discuss its application in health-care. This paragraph need not be overly technical, since it is not a research assignment.

Ultrasound

This is a fairly recent technology. With this invention, certain tests are affordable and practical for both the patient and the practitioner. Ultrasound has different velocities these differ in density and elasticity with different tissues. Ultrasound is a technique that has changed medicine. Ultrasound transmits sound waves through body tissues and records the echoes as the sounds encounter other objects within the body. The use of ultrasound is noninvasive. Ultrasound can be used to measure the size and shape of some internal organs. It is commonly used for monitoring fetuses. Ultrasound can detect abnormalities. Ultrasound is painless. Ultrasound does not harm the internal organs or a fetus. Ultrasound is also used in physical therapy. It has been know to help circulation and regeneration of tissue. Ultrasound requires specialized equipment but it can be used in a variety of ways.

UNIT EXTENSIONS

1. Go to a writing website and locate information on a health career of your choice. Draft one paragraph detailing the information you located on the Internet.

2. Go to a store that specializes in vitamins and supplements. Get some advice on improving your diet. Write a paragraph that includes the information you received and whether or not you agree with it.

3. Write an opinion paragraph on one healthcare concern or issue in your community.

UNIT 7 SELF-CHECK

1. Draw a sketch of a well-developed paragraph. Label the three important parts and any distinguishing features that a paragraph should have.

2. Imagine you are in a test situation. Relying on the information you have today and your personal experiences in healthcare, select <u>one</u> of the topics below and write a paragraph. Ensure varied sentence structure and adequate support.

   a. November 14, 1666, is the recorded date of the first blood transfusion. Samuel Pepys of London, England, recorded the event in his diary. There have been many changes and advances in medical treatment since that day. Select one medical breakthrough and discuss its impact on healthcare.

   b. Consider your lifestyle and diet in relationship to your overall health. Select two ways by which you could improve your health. Provide rationale and support for selecting these two specific improvements.

3. In a previous assignment, students were asked to write on this topic: *How does one ensure a healthy diet?* Read the sentences provided below (a, b, c, and d).
   Assemble the sentences (a, b, c, and d) into a well-rounded paragraph. You may add, delete, or change any part of these sentences as you draft your paragraph.

   a. To ensure a healthy diet, one should increase his or her dietary fiber; therefore, eating at least five servings of fruits and vegetables a day is important.

   b. Along with five servings of fruit and vegetables, one should add whole grains and beans to achieve a healthy diet.

   c. A diet that consists of foods low in saturated fats will help ensure low cholesterol.

   d. Eating a well-balanced diet will provide you with adequate vitamins and nutrients; therefore, it will help create a healthier person.

(Original paragraph assignment submitted by a student, Tina Horner.)

UNIT 8

Writing Skills with Definition

UNIT TERMS

Concluding sentence	A sentence that helps bring the paragraph to a close
Indentation	One tab or about five single spaces at the beginning of a paragraph
Support sentence	A sentence that supports the topic sentence
Topic sentence	Also called the main-idea sentence; provides the central idea and direction to the paragraph
Transition word	A word or group of words that helps join ideas or sentences
Definition paragraph	A paragraph that defines a term

UNIT OBJECTIVES

Upon completion of this unit, the student will be able to

1. recognize the parts of a definition

2. draft a definition sentence that is effective

3. draft paragraphs using text question prompts

4. revise and improve definitions that are sentences and paragraphs

Glossary of Medical Terms

Term	Part of Speech	Definition
allograft	noun	transplant tissue
arrhythmia	noun	irregular heartbeat
atrium	noun	upper chamber of each half of the heart
autoimmune disease	noun	a disease that occurs when the body no longer tolerates its own antigenic markers on cells
biopsy	noun	the removal of a tissue sample for study
cecum	noun	the first part of the large intestine
computed tomography scan (CT)	noun	a radiographic technique that selects a body section and allows a clear view of the selected anatomy
congenital	adjective	present at birth
conjunctivitis	noun	inflammation of the conjunctiva of the eye
diverticulitis	noun	inflammation of the diverticula in the intestine
dyspnea	noun	difficulty in breathing

dysphagia	noun	inability or difficulty in swallowing
epistaxis	noun	nosebleed; hemorrhage of the nose
exacerbation	noun	a worsening of a condition
fulguration	noun	destruction of tissue by electric sparks
gastroscopy	noun	examination of the stomach and abdominal cavity
lactose intolerance	noun	an inability of digest milk and other dairy products
latent	adjective	not active; hidden
polyp	noun	a tumor with a footlike structure
radiographic	adjective	a process of obtaining an image with X-rays
remission	noun	a lessening of severity or a period with no symptoms of illness
scabies	noun	a highly communicable disease causes by an itch mite
splenography	noun	a record or description of the spleen
stridor	noun	a harsh high-pitched sound heard during respiration
ventricles	noun	the two lower chambers of the heart
venule	noun	a small vein

DEFINITION SENTENCES

The three parts of a formal definition are the term, the formal group or class it belongs to, and the term's distinguishing features. The distinguishing features should separate the term from all other words in the class; these features make that specific word unique.

Term	Class or Group	Distinguishing Features
biopsy	surgical procedure	used to obtain a representative tissue sample for microscopic examination to establish a diagnosis
allograft	surgical procedure	used to transplant skin from the same species

To write a definition sentence, combine the three parts into a grammatical sentence:

A biopsy is a surgical procedure that is used to obtain a representative tissue sample for microscopic examination, which will help establish a diagnosis.

An allograft is a surgical procedure that transplants skin from like species.

Adding an appositive phrase to a simple sentence can further provide a definition that assists the writer in showing the depth of knowledge:

Computed tomography (CT) scan, a variation of the radiographic technique, is a diagnostic imaging technique used in detecting soft body tissue diseases.

There are primarily two methods used to define terms or procedures in healthcare, text-based definitions and definitions set off by punctuation.

WORD CLUES INDICATING DEFINITION

First are text-based word clues such as *is, was, are, means, also known as, involves, is called, or, defined as, that is, serves as, refers to,* or *resembles*. For example:

The cecum is the first two or three inches of the large intestine.

Jaundice, also known as icterus, is a yellowing of the skin and one of the symptoms of several liver disorders.

Autoimmune diseases have flare-ups or exacerbations and remissions or latent periods.

PUNCTUATION INDICATING DEFINITIONS

And second, punctuation often sets off definitions. These punctuation symbols include commas, parentheses, and dashes. These are very helpful for learning the synonyms and definitions for medical terms. Often a medical term has a common or popular term that is used and is familiar to most people, and this term may be given inside specific punctuation marks. For example:

Conjunctivitis, pinkeye, is an inflammation of the membrane that lines the eyelid and the surface of the eye.

Scabs (crustations) may form over sores and wounds.

Venules, little veins, are formed from the union of capillaries.

Sterile technique—also called reverse isolation technique—is used to care for the patient.

EXERCISE 8-1: Complete the chart for the medical terms below. You might need a medical dictionary. These terms will be used later in this unit.

Term	Class/Group	Distinguishing Features
polyp		
gastroscopy		
scabies		
fulguration		
dyspnea		
epistaxis		
arrhythmia		

(continued)

Term	Class/Group	Distinguishing Features
stridor		
splenography		
dysphagia		

Exercise 8-2: Draft sentences for the above terms that use word clues as a means of signaling definition.

1. polyp

____

____

2. gastroscopy

____

____

3. scabies

____

____

4. fulguration

____

____

5. dyspnea

____

____

6. epistaxis

____

____

7. arrhythmia

____

____

8. stridor

____

____

9. splenography

____

____

10. dysphagia

____

____

Sometimes defining a term is as simple as providing a synonym. In this case, the term is usually given followed by *is, are, means, refers to, defined as,* or the like, and then the synonym is provided. Avoid using the term or a derivative of it as part of the definition. For example:

Anacusis is deafness.

Strep throat is a sore throat caused by streptococcal bacteria.

THE DEFINITION PARAGRAPH

Sometimes a single sentence definition may not provide the complete answer, so this calls for an expanded definition. The entire paragraph develops the definition of the term or concept. In healthcare, we often need to explain the specific details of a condition or situation in order to ensure accuracy, so a paragraph may be necessary to provide the complete definition. Definition paragraphs can use a variety of techniques to provide the meaning of the term or concept. Writers can use a formal definition, synonyms, antonyms, etymology, and detailed explanations.

A definition paragraph usually begins with a topic sentence that provides the one term or phrase term being defined. The topic sentence should include one of the terms indicating that a definition is being given:

Definition Signal Words			
is	is called	serves as	is known as
are	is defined as	is referred to as	means
also known as	that is	which means	resembles

A writer can use the three formal parts of a definition to draft a topic sentence.

Term	Class/Group	Distinguishing Features
diverticulitis	diverticular disease	*Inflammation in the small pouches of the weakened intestinal walls.*

For example:

Diverticulitis is the inflammatory disease of the diverticula, which are small pouches in weakened intestinal walls.

Such a sentence helps establish the controlling idea and terms of the paragraph. The reader has a definite sense that the paragraph will cover the definition of *diverticulitis.* The topic sentence or main-idea sentence should state what is being defined and provide its classification. This is often similar to the single-sentence definitions that were practiced earlier in this unit. This sentence will control the type of definition to be provided and the level of detail.

Supporting sentences will continue to develop the definition. The definition is developed by limiting the information in the paragraph to only that information that supports the term being developed. If not enough detail is given in the support sentences, then the definition of the term or concept becomes vague or even undefined. Phrases that may direct and assist the reader in understanding that a definition is being given are terms like _____ *can be defined as* or _____ *can be considered,* _____ *means that,* or *to define* _____. This paragraph will include the term parts of a definition: the term, the class or group, and the distinguishing features of the term. In the example of *diverticulitis,* the support sentences might be

> *These pouches are most likely to occur in the colon. This disease results from feces and bacteria, which are trapped in these weakened pouches. The initial onset of the disease may take several years, or it may come in the form of a sudden attack. Symptoms of diverticulitis include fever, abdominal pain and tenderness, and a general feeling of discomfort. Treatment for mild cases is antibiotics and changes in the diet. If perforation of the intestinal wall occurs, surgery is necessary. Interestingly, a diet high in fiber is considered the most important step in the prevention of diverticulitis.*

Word choice continues to be important; the use of synonyms will be important in expressing the term's features or specific characteristics. In a definition paragraph, examples may be used to develop the definition. Choose the specific examples, facts, and/or incidents to illustrate your definition. What information you ultimately include in the definition paragraph will reflect your depth of understanding, judgment, and point of view, so the selection of this information is important to the success of your paragraph. Avoid making generalizations; after all, the purpose of a definition is to provide specifics about a term, condition, or procedure in healthcare.

The concluding sentence brings the paragraph to a close by signaling the final part of the definition and is generally tied to a larger context or application. It signals the end of the definition. The information from the paragraph should be summarized in a meaningful way:

> *Although diverticulitis can be painful and medical treatment may be needed along with dietary changes, the prognosis for a complete recovery is excellent.*

Thus, the completed definition paragraph is as follows:

> *Diverticulitis is the inflammation of the diverticula, which are small pouches in weakened intestinal walls. These pouches are most likely to occur in the colon. This disease results from feces and bacteria, which are trapped in these weakened*

pouches. The initial onset of the disease may take several years, or it may come in the form of a sudden attack. Symptoms of diverticulitis include fever, abdominal pain and tenderness, and a general feeling of discomfort. Treatment for mild cases is antibiotics and changes in diet. If perforation of the intestinal wall occurs, surgery is necessary. Interestingly, a diet high in fiber is considered the most important step in the prevention of diverticulitis. Although diverticulitis can be painful and medical treatment may be needed along with dietary changes, the prognosis for a complete recovery is excellent.

EXERCISE 8-3: Read the sentences below. Determine each sentence's purpose in the paragraph and label as follows: topic sentence *(TS)*, supporting sentence *(SS)*, or concluding sentence *(CS)*.

1. ______ *In summary, the cardiac cycle is the sequence that keeps blood moving from the veins, through the heart, into the arteries, and through the body.*
2. ______ *Studies have shown that lactase deficiency may be congenital, resulting from prematurity, or it may be acquired.*
3. ______ *Thus, lactose intolerance may be controlled by modifying the diet or taking medication.*
4. ______ *The cardiac cycle is the sequence of events that occur in one heartbeat.*
5. ______ *Next, the atria, upper heart chambers receiving venous blood, relax, and the ventricles, lower heart chambers pumping blood to the body, contract.*
6. ______ *Pneumonia is a bacterial infection of the lungs.*
7. ______ *Lactose intolerance is the inability to digest lactose resulting from the deficiency of the enzyme lactase.*
8. ______ *Many bacteria can cause pneumonia; streptococcus pneumoniae is the most common cause.*

EXERCISE 8-4: Write a definition paragraph. Choose one of the following terms or concepts and define it in a paragraph. You will need to rely on the Internet or other reference materials to locate information.

- **a.** Alzheimer's disease
- **b.** Maslow's theory
- **c.** Glaucoma
- **d.** Botulism
- **e.** Fetal alcohol syndrome
- **f.** Any topic approved by your instructor

Use the checklist to ensure that your definition paragraph contains the essential features of a definition paragraph.

Definition Paragraph Checklist

Check the following boxes:

☐ Yes	☐ No	Is the term mentioned in the topic sentence?
☐ Yes	☐ No	Is the class or group mentioned in the topic sentence?
☐ Yes	☐ No	Are the distinguishing features in the topic sentence?
☐ Yes	☐ No	Do the support sentences further define the distinguishing features?
☐ Yes	☐ No	Are the support sentences adequate to define the term effectively?
☐ Yes	☐ No	Do transition words help unite the sentences and aid the reader in understanding the paragraph?
☐ Yes	☐ No	Is there a concluding sentence?
☐ Yes	☐ No	Does the concluding sentence draw the paragraph to a meaningful close?
☐ Yes	☐ No	Has a spelling check been done?
☐ Yes	☐ No	Are the sentences varied in length and content?
☐ Yes	☐ No	Are the sentences punctuated correctly?
☐ Yes	☐ No	Do subjects and verbs agree?

DEFINITION QUESTIONS ON EXAMS

Recognizing definition questions on tests is important because then you will know what information the answer should include. Definition questions usually include words such as *means, involves, is called, that is, which means, resembles*, or *defined as*. Some examples are

1. Define the term aneurysm.

2. What is the Valsalva's maneuver?

3. Explain what ___________ is.

It is important to answer these types of questions in a complete sentence. For example, *Define the term aneurysm.* The answer would be

An aneurysm is a diagnostic term for the localized abnormal dilation of a vessel or artery that results in a rupture.

UNIT PROOFREADING EXERCISES

Proofread the following paragraph. Locate and change any errors in grammar, usage, sentence structure, and punctuation.

Quitting smoking is one of the most important things you can do for you health. There is a lot of methods to help smoker quit. One method is the nicotine patch. They are patches that release nicotine into the bloodstream in through the skin. The patch helps some smokers gradually withdraw from the nicotine addict. it is one method that help smokers who have the withdrawal symptoms of headaches anxiety depression and insomnia. By combining the patch and a smoking cessation program a smoker chances for success can be increased.

UNIT REVISION EXERCISES

The paragraph below has many problems. Some sentences are awkward; others are out of order. Some sentences are run on, while others may be fragments. Revise this definition paragraph so that it is a good example of a definition paragraph. Use the checklist presented in this unit to ensure an effective paragraph.

The test for TB includes a skin test. Also saliva sample and a chest X-ray. It is called TB. Others inhale the bacteria. Sometimes it takes up to two years for a person to develop active TB. When people with TB cough or sneeze the infected bacteria become airborne. Tuberculosis is a contagious disease. It is caused by bacteria that infects the lungs. Others never do. Active TB is known for having the symptoms of weight lost, fatigue, fever, persistent cough, and general malaise. They create small areas of inflammation. Drug treatment for active treatment of TB is available it may take 6 to 12 months to cure. If not treated a person can die from TB. It can spread to other body parts. Especially to the brain, kidneys, and bones. The bacteria multiply.

UNIT EXTENSIONS

1. Write a definition paragraph that defines *spherical power* and *cylinder power*.
2. Write a definition paragraph defining *well-being*.
3. Define *public health* in a paragraph.

UNIT 8 SELF-CHECK

1. What are the three parts of a formal definition sentence or paragraph?

   a. ______________________

b. ______________________________

c. ______________________________

2. You may use a medical dictionary. Write a sentence definition for:

   a. comedo

   ____

   ____

   ____

   ____

   b. pediculosis

   ____

   ____

   ____

   ____

3. Choose one of the terms below. Draft a definition paragraph of your own. You may use any reference books you choose to gather your notes. This paragraph needs to be your own definition of the term. Use the definition checklist to assist you in editing the paragraph.

   a. atherosclerosis
   b. chlamydia
   c. macular degeneration
   d. sinusitis
   e. bursitis

UNIT 9

Writing Skills with Summaries

UNIT TERMS

Cliché	An overused phrase that is no longer meaningful
Cover letter	A letter that accompanies a job application and resumé
Paraphrase	To restate in your own words information written by another writer
Resumé	A summary of your qualifications for a specific position
Summary	The main ideas capturing the key points of an article, chapter, or concept
Thank-you note	A brief letter or note that is appreciative of some opportunity

UNIT OBJECTIVES

Upon completion of this unit, the student will be able to

1. define paraphrasing
2. define summarizing
3. use summary skills to assist in completing job applications
4. draft a summary paragraph using paraphrasing and summarizing skills
5. apply writing skills to business writing needs
6. draft a resumé
7. draft a cover letter
8. draft a thank-you note

Glossary of Medical Terms

Term	Part of Speech	Definition
acute	adjective	severe, sharp, occurring quickly
chronic	adjective	of long duration
diabetic	noun; adjective	a person who has diabetes, a chronic carbohydrate metabolism disorder that results from a lack of or an inadequate production of insulin; also, an adjective describing this condition

epistaxis	noun	nosebleed
glucose	noun	sugar or dextrose
lice	noun	plural of louse, a small insect that lives off humans or other animals
limb	noun	an arm or a leg
nit	noun	the egg of a louse
peripheral nerves	adjective	nerves away from the center of the body, as in the legs and feet
pediculosis	noun	infestation with lice
transient	adjective	changing; without a home
ulcerate	verb	to cause or to develop an ulcer

Summarizing is an important writing skill. Summarizing is a process of restating a passage or thoughts in your own words so that they reflect the original information. When you read a passage or take notes, those notes are a summary of the main ideas and important points from the reading. Most important in a summary is to provide the most critical or important points. To do this requires the ability to distinguish between main ideas and supporting ideas. In addition, you need to know how to paraphrase. Summarizing captures the main idea of an article, chapter, or concept. Putting the main idea of these in your own words, or paraphrasing, allows you to learn the concepts and facts more readily.

A practical application of summarizing is the resumé. A resumé is a summary of your specific work experiences in response to a job description or objective. The selection of the words to describe your experiences is critical. You need to use the language of the profession and provide an illustration of your skills in words. Examples of these summaries associated with work applications include questions like:

1. What makes you qualified for this position?
2. Why does this job appeal to you?
3. Explain any skills unique to your application.
4. How did you learn of this position?

PARAPHRASING

Paraphrasing is restating the information you have read or heard in your own words and way. To accurately paraphrase may require you to read the article or paragraph several times to completely understand it. One technique that helps students to accomplish this is: Read the paragraph or article several times. Then close your eyes and orally restate the main idea of the passage. When you do this, it will be in your own words because usually the ideas are too complex to memorize in several readings. Then, write what you have orally stated. Check it against the reading passage to ensure that you have correctly represented the information and that you have used your own words.

SUMMARY SENTENCES

Summary sentences are often used to restate the main idea of a paragraph or article. These types of sentences show your understanding of the purpose of the paragraph or article. You have to be able to take many ideas and make one sentence that expresses one main idea. Although the information has been condensed, you must keep its overall meaning.

Identifying the source by providing the author and the title of the material is important to ensure accuracy and traceability. A variety of introductory phrases may be used to accomplish recognizing the source of the information. Giving credit to the proper source is part of being a professional and is easy to accomplish.

You can use the following phrases to set up a summary sentence by simply adding in the author's name and the article or text's title. Note that these are summary sentences, so their quotes are indirect, or paraphrased. Quotation marks are used around the exact words of another author. For example,

(The author) notes in (this article) that . . .

(The author) in (this article) shows that . . .

In (this article) (the author) writes that . . .

As (the author) states in (this article) . . .

As shown by (the author) in (this article) . . .

The main point (the author) makes in (the article) is

Summary sentences need strong verbs to introduce and reflect the author's main points. For example: *The main point Brown is saying is that an adequate source of B vitamins needs to be found (weak construction). Brown points out the need for better sources of Vitamin B (stronger construction).*

Many strong verbs are available to choose from; some are provided below:

advises	establishes	points out
argues	explains	proposes
asks	expounds	recommends
asserts	finds	reviews
believes	implies	reveals
claims	insists	shows
contends	maintains	states
declares	notes	suggests

When you use another writer's ideas, be accurate and document the source of your information. Article titles within a text are placed in quotations; book, journal, and newspaper titles are in italics or underlined.

Here are some examples of summary sentences:

1. *So, as Brown states in "The Amazing Human Cell," each type of human cell functions in a group, not individually, and contributes to the human body.*
2. *In summary, the nervous system regulates our activities, simple to complex.*
3. *Thus, one can conclude that proper blood circulation is totally dependent on the proper functioning of the heart.*

EXERCISE 9-1: Read the passages below and then write a summary sentence for each, capturing the main idea of the passage.

Diabetics often have problems with their feet. One reason is that the peripheral nerves are damaged by poor circulation. The legs and feet are often affected because these are farthest from the heart's action; thus, blood circulation may be limited. Furthermore, abnormal blood glucose levels can damage blood vessels and nerves that take nourishment and nerve signals to the legs and feet. This damage then leads to the limbs becoming numb, feeling less pain, and having difficulty healing. With the loss of sensation, an individual may be unaware of foot sores or injuries. The feet then become ulcerated and infected. So, limb and foot care are important to maintain proper circulation and foot health.

Summary sentence:

____

____

____

Pain is an alarm system that gets our attention. Pain can signal that something has gone wrong with our bodies. It is a basic symptom of inflammation and can help an individual figure out what is wrong with his or her body. Pain comes in various sensations: throbbing, stabbing, or aching. Pain may be localized or generalized. Pain can be acute or chronic in nature. Furthermore, it can be mild or severe. Pain works as a help signal to pay attention to our bodies.

Summary sentence:

____

____

____

Nosebleeds (epistaxis) are common occurrences. When the tiny capillaries inside the nose rupture, a nosebleed occurs. A nosebleed can be caused by simply blowing one's nose, having a cold or an allergy, being in cold or extremely hot and dry weather, or being hit in the face or nose. Usually pain does not accompany a nosebleed. Nosebleeds may have a small trickle of blood or produce severe and sudden bleeding. Nosebleeds are usually handled by first aid at home. So, although a nosebleed can be unsettling, usually it is nothing severe and can be managed by home care.

Summary sentence:

____

____

____

SUMMARY PARAGRAPHS

Summary paragraphs are used to provide more detailed information than a summary sentence. The paragraph follows the paragraph format and often can use a summary sentence as its main-idea sentence. This type of paragraph is often used to demonstrate a cumulative skill or knowledge, as in the following assignments:

1. *Summarize your learning curve during this clinical rotation. What did you learn about yourself during this course?*
2. *Summarize your understanding of Maslow's theory as it applies to the homeless or transient populations.*

You may be asked to summarize an article or theory. To accomplish this, break the task into several steps:

1. Read the article or theory and then use your paraphrasing skills to restate the main idea in your own words. Consider what the author's point is and what he or she wants you to understand from the reading of the article.
2. Draft a main-idea sentence. If the author presents new information or a unique point of view, it is important to use the author's name and source. The main-idea sentence should be clear and concise.
3. Select the most important details to support the main-idea sentence. Specific examples may be cited, or you may relate your own experience to the ideas from the passage. Key to the success of the support sentences is that they support in example and words the ideas of the main-idea sentence. A common error is that students select examples or the details that contradict the main point. Avoid trying to include every detail the author used. Select the most pertinent ones. Use your own words, not the author's words. Give credit to the original author by citing the source.

4. Write a concluding sentence that shows the relevance of the article or the main idea to your task, your career, or your specific learning objectives. You may express a new concept you have learned or a fresh perspective to something you have learned before. This demonstrates to the reader that you have insight from the reading.

Concluding phrases may be helpful in drawing the summary paragraph to a close. Experiment with a wide variety of these phrases to add to your sentence variety:

For the reasons above	To sum up	In review
As noted	In summation	Concluding
In conclusion	In other words	In short
Without a doubt	In brief	Summarizing

EXERCISE 9-2: Choose one of the assignments below to complete.

1. Locate an article in a news magazine such as *Time* and *Newsweek;* both have articles on health, science, and medical issues. Draft a summary sentence first, then write a summary paragraph. Include a citation of source.

2. Select a journal in your specific healthcare field. Read the article several times and look up any new terminology. Then draft a summary main-idea sentence and write a summary paragraph of the article.

SUMMARY SKILLS ON JOB APPLICATIONS

Much of the writing done for job applications requires skills in summarizing. All of the information on the job application and in the cover letter and resumé need to market your strengths. This information must be an accurate representation of your strengths and abilities. All of the information should match.

Language should always be professional in a job application or correspondence. Avoid clichéd or overused spoken forms. Oral language forms or overused phrases detract from the professional tone.

JOB APPLICATIONS

Job applications may be submitted electronically or in handwritten form. Most important is that the applicant follows these basics:

1. Read through the application first so that you can plan what information you need to place in the separate section. This avoids repeating the same information in several places.

2. Read the directions carefully so that the information is placed in the correct location.

3. Be prepared to fill out the application if you complete the application on site. Perhaps it is better to ask to take the application with you and complete it at home.

4. Ensure that the data you will fill out matches your resumé and is factual.
5. Spelling does count. Neatness is critical. Use dark pen.
6. Summary sentences need to be polished and informative. These must answer the question directly.
7. The information presented should help separate you from other applicants.
8. Match the skills that you possess with those that the employer is seeking.
9. Do not leave any spaces blank.
10. Have someone proofread your application if possible.

Most organizations have their own applications and processes for applying for a position. The key is to *proofread* everything prior to submission, be neat and accurate in the information presented, and keep a *copy* for your records.

Remember that the application itself may get you an interview. So attention to detail is critical:

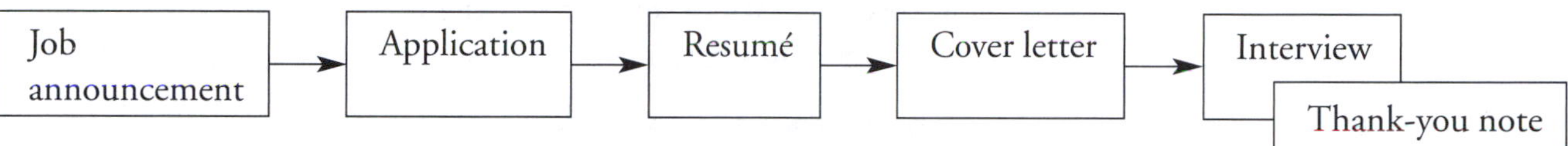

RESUMÉS

A resumé is a summary of your specific work experiences and qualifications in response to a job description or objective. The selection of the words to describe your experiences is critical. There is no one correct format for a resumé. A resumé reflects a person's perception of his or her abilities and qualifications. Use the language of the profession and provide an illustration in print of your background and depth of experience. To be responsive to a job posting, a person should tailor his or her skills into a summary that highlights the skills needed to perform the specific job. Key is the selection of specific strong verbs that capture skills, especially because phrases, not sentences, are used to describe experience. The point of a resumé is to illustrate in words what the individual is bringing to the position.

The layout and organization of your resumé either adds to or detracts from your information. It is important to realize that the resumé should be organized so that it is clear what your skills are and how they specifically meet the job requirements of the position that you are applying for. The major sections of the resumé are typically include

1. Your personal information: name, address, contact information
2. An objective only if there is a clear target and a specific employment goal that is sought. Objectives are not as popular as they once were. Use with a very specific job target.
3. Work experience, including places of employment, dates, and the skills that you developed while being employed
4. Education, formal and informal, as well as any certificates or specialized training

5. Volunteer work or community involvement, if applicable
6. Specialized information such as professional memberships, honors, awards, and the like

It is important to place the most important information at the top of your resumé. This allows the prospective employer to review that information first. Present the information with the most information first, followed by subsequent information. Each section should present the information in this order.

Other helpful hints:

- Be truthful.
- Limit the resumé to one or two pages depending experience and qualifications.
- Use headings consistently. Try to limit the font types and sizes to two. This allows for a professional look to the resumé.
- Empty spaces or "white space" helps the reader locate and focus on the most important information.
- Match your skills with those needed for the position.
- Never overfill or stuff a resumé full of minute details that do not relate to the position sought.
- Limit adjectives; use strong verbs.
- Keep language simple and direct.
- The information under the heading must provide specific detail about what the heading claims it to be.
- Use bullets or indentations to help separate information.
- Do be professional; avoid overpersonalization of the information.
- References belong on the application form, not on the resumé.

There are three types of resumés: chronological, functional, and targeted. The type of resumé selected depends on the experience of the individual:

Type of resume	Use in these situations or conditions
Chronological	• with a stable work history • when work experience is in a logical progression to current position being sought • to put most current experience first in order—not using a historical time order
Functional	• to focus on skills rather than the time and place of employment • for an individual who has been studying, not working • for an individual who has not been employed recently to highlight skills • for an individual who is changing careers

Targeted	• to highlight the specific capabilities possessed as related to the position being sought • to focus on past work experience • when the current job is not directly related to the position being sought

Sample resumes follow.

Chronological Sample Resumé

Mary K. Browne
431287 17th Street
Seattle, WA 98012
(206) 555-0100
MaryKBrown@hotmail.com

WORK EXPERIENCE

Valley Health Villa, Seattle, WA 1999–present

Lead Certified Nursing Assistant

- Mentor new certified nursing assistants in facility policies and procedures
- Oversee the resident–new employee relations
- Provide patient care to residents, day shift
- Promote tactile and sensory recreational techniques
- Host monthly family gatherings
- Edit and publish monthly residents' newsletter

Meadows Skilled Nursing Facility, Seattle, WA 1992–1999

Certified Nursing Assistant

- Provided daily patient care to 8–15 residents
- Encouraged resident self-care
- Documented activities in a timely fashion and as required
- Coordinated with nursing and families to ensure patient comfort and wellness
- Attended healthcare training: Healing Touch, HIV/AIDS Procedures and Handling Grief; CPR

Activities Coordinator 1990–1992

- Provided individual recreational activities for residents: puzzles, books and magazines, sewing projects, crafts, painting, drawing, and computer training
- Developed group activities for 180 residents: movie night, dances, holiday socials, craft fairs, discussion groups, outings to local activities
- Ensured each resident had an activity plan documented in his or her record meeting facility and state requirements for social activities
- Coordinated with nursing staff and administration to ensure safe and appropriate social activities

EDUCATION

Certified Nursing Assistant Training, Renton Technical College 1992

Functional Sample Resumé

Sandy McCallie
3452 Washington Road
Anacortes, WA 98221
(360) 555-0100
believenself@yahoo.com

Supervisory/Management

- Responsible for preparing and implementing in-service for all new healthcare team members
- Contribute to the in-service program offered to all staff twice a year
- Lead nursing team providing optimum healthcare
- Participate in the interview process of new staff
- Attend state and national meetings to track and maintain the latest in healthcare policy, procedures, and patient care
- Coordinate medical procedure training with the practicing doctors

Public Relations

- Conduct training sessions for conflict resolution
- Offer three courses in grieving and handling loss through illness
- Encourage excellence in patient and family relationships with staff
- Serve as advisor to the hospital administrator
- Educate the public about changes occurring within the hospital
- Host a *Get to Know Your Healthcare Center*

Community Activism

- Promotion of health fairs in public schools, local library, and senior centers
- Lead cancer fundraising efforts in community
- Represent senior citizens in local and regional policy making meetings
- Hospice volunteer
- Member of the local Red Cross

EMPLOYMENT HISTORY

1988–present **Anacortes Hospital**
Head Nurse and Supervisor of Healthcare Team

1986–1988 **Highlands Villa**
Night Supervisor, Head Nurse

Targeted Sample Resumé

Bob R. Smith
345 Cedar Street
Berkeley, CA
(501) 555-0100
Healthy1@hotmail.com

CAPABILITIES

- Develop and publish a newsletter
- Design and implement a website

- Plan and draft manuals and policy handbooks
- Handle high-pressure publishing deadlines
- Specialize in clear communication and technical writing

ACHIEVEMENTS
- Received commendations for working with healthcare companies to publish accurate and timely information
- Publish several how-to manuals for administration and staff
- Supervised staff to ensure publication quality and deadlines

COMPUTER EXPERIENCE

Internet	email, Netscape, Internet Explorer, HTML
Word Processing	Word 2003, WordPerfect
Hardware	PC and Macs
Desktop Publishing	Publisher, Pagemaker
Spreadsheets/Database	Excel, Access

WORK HISTORY

2000–Present	Tang Medical Center Public Relations Director
1998–2000	Health for the City Writer and Public Speaker

EDUCATION
- University of California, Berkeley; B.A. in Public Health

References and Portfolio Available Upon Request

Resumés must make it easy for the reader to locate the information. Writers need to keep in mind that the resumé will get a "10-second read," so the resumé must be clear, focused, and appropriate to the position it is responding to. One way to accomplish this is by headings and bullets. An applicant can use headings and spacing to highlight appropriate information.

For example, suppose the job posting reads:

Needed: Experienced registered nurse to provide care to home-bound terminally ill patient.

An appropriate heading on the responding resumé might be:

Home Healthcare Provider
- Skilled in hospice care for acutely, chronically, or terminally ill individuals
- Experienced in locating and working with appropriate local healthcare service providers, collaborating with families and other service providers
- Provided fifteen years of hospital care-giving experience as a registered nurse at Regional Medical Hospital in acute and trauma care section

In developing descriptive phrases, use strong verbs that illustrate your abilities and the transferable skills that you possess. Transferable skills are those skills that have multiple applications; these add value to an application. Look at the table of transferable skills below. These are the transferable skills of a certified nursing assistant who has worked for a long-term care facility for two years.

People Skills	Patient Care	Leadership	Recordkeeping
diplomatic	diligent	good at listening	neat and tidy
skilled at negotiating	concerned	able to delegate	accurate
high-energy	supportive	able to make decisions	good at communicating
adaptable	patient	responsible	detail-oriented
team player	conscientious	punctual	analytical
sensitive	trustworthy	safety-conscious	honest
bilingual	respectful	results-oriented	independent

Notice that the skills cited by the individual in the example above also probably match the work expectations of the facility where she works. Such a table can help a job seeker communicate the skills that he or she has. These terms help a person answer the employer's primary question, "Why should I hire you?"

EXERCISE 9-3: Consider the skills that you have gained from work and college. Then develop a table of transferable skills.

People Skills	Patient Care	Leadership	Recordkeeping

A second helpful hint is to use varied and strong verbs to describe your skills and qualifications through the previous work experience.

achieved	directed	organized	***Add your own***
advised	equipped	performed	________
analyzed	established	persuaded	________
assisted	evaluated	planned	________
completed	expanded	processed	________

coordinated	generated	produced	________
counseled	handled	served	________
created	initiated	set up	________
delivered	led	taught	________
developed	managed	wrote	________

EXERCISE 9-4: Using the words in the table above, draft a sample resumé highlighting your specific skills to a job opening in your field. Use the commercially available resumé software to format your prose. Draft a resumé in any of these styles that markets your skills.

COVER LETTERS

Cover letters are helpful documents because they can serve several purposes: These letters can differentiate one candidate from and other, and they can draw attention to your specific strengths that appear elsewhere, such as in the application or on your resumé.

A cover letter needs to accomplish three things:

1. show why the employer should consider you
2. summarize your key qualifications
3. illustrate your professionalism

The style and the content of the cover letter should be appropriate for the position you desire. Writers should avoid a writing style that attempts to impress; instead, the writer needs to present his or her content so that the content and organization impresses the reader. By following some simple guidelines, writers can write a clear and effective cover letter:

1. Begin the letter with a clear sentence that indicates the job you are applying for. Note why you want this specific position and how you learned about the opening.
2. Clearly state you how your specific experience differentiates you from other candidates. Focus on specific attributes you can contribute.
3. Mention any relevant special training that will make you the right choice. Most people applying for the post will have similar educations, so just noting your degrees is not enough.
4. End in a professional yet cordial close. Avoid clichéd endings: *Thank you for your consideration.* Use some other close that separates you from others, such as noting your interest in the position or your availability for a phone conversation.
5. Make every sentence count. A sentence such as "I have been looking for a challenging job for a long time" is not effective. Write sentences that will have an impact on the reader.

An effective letter will get to the point quickly, summarize your top qualifications, highlight your specific interest in the post, and demonstrate something about your professionalism and personality. A one-page cover letter should accomplish this so that the letter remains concise and clear.

Sample Cover Letter

12987 17th Avenue
Bershire, CA 89762
March 21, 2005

Carol Moss
Nature's Bend Retirement Center
45 North Road
Yelstone, CA 89762

Dear Ms. Moss:

I would like to apply for the position of certified nursing assistant as posited in the Yelstone Times on March 20, 2005.

Enclosed please find my resumé, detailing my specialized training and work experience. Of interest may be my bilingual abilities in Chinese and my specialized training. I have attended several recent training sessions that promote healing touch and sensory training for Alzheimer's patients:

- Healing Touch Conference: focused on caregivers' touch to assist patients in feeling secure and in their sense of well-being (February 2005)
- Keeping Patients Secure: tailored to assisting the needs of Alzheimer's patients' sense of security and ways to ensure patient safety (December 2004)
- Educating the Whole Family: provided information on how to communicate with patient families within the confines of patient confidentiality and site policy

I am interested in working at Nature's Bend because I have visited several friends and relatives at your facility. Impressed with the high quality of care and the friendly staff, I am inspired to seek employment at your facility.

I look forward to an opportunity to interview for this position. Please telephone me at 206-555-0100.

Sincerely,

Ivy Lazare

Enclosure

Exercise 9-5: Draft a cover letter that applies for a position and that includes key elements of your resumé and transferable skills list.

THANK-YOU NOTES

A friendly letter is a good way to illustrate your professionalism. It is appropriate to send a thank-you note for an interview, to a person who has been a reference for a job application, and for other professional assistance that an individual receives. In general, a thank-you note follows the same general format as the cover letter. Use professional language and ensure that the names and dates referred to in the thank-you are correct:

> 12987 17th Avenue
> Bershire, CA 89762
> March 21, 2005
>
> Carol Moss
> Nature's Bend Retirement Center
> 45 North Road
> Yelstone, CA 89762
>
> Dear Ms. Moss:
>
> Thank you for interviewing me for the position of Certified Nursing Assistant at Nature's Bend. I appreciated the tour and the introduction to the Nature's Bend staff.
>
> I look forward to hearing your decision. Please telephone me at 206-555-0100. I am available to begin orientation immediately.
>
> Sincerely,
>
> Ivy Lazare

Sometimes students ask what to include in a professional thank-you note. Include the names of the individuals who participated in the interview, the date, and the position or title that you interviewed for. Sometimes it is important to mention something about the questions asked or how helpful the interviewer was in answering your questions. Always end with a contact number and a professional closing.

Computer skills are workplace skills. Type all correspondence to any potential employer.

EXERCISE 9-6: Draft a sample thank-you note that is a follow-up to the cover letter and interview process.

Job Applications Checklists

Cover Letter

- ☐ Correct name of addressee and addresses
- ☐ Mention of where you learned of the position and the position applied for

- ☐ Your interest in position with that specific company (you want the position)
- ☐ A summary of your skills for the specific position
- ☐ A brief summary of your experience relevant to the position
- ☐ A statement of why this position is for you (you can do the job)
- ☐ Note of your desire for an interview
- ☐ A way to contact you
- ☐ A professional appearance of the cover letter
- ☐ Professional language

Resumé

- ☐ Correct name and contact information for you
- ☐ A stated objective that is specific to the position you are applying for
- ☐ Focus on skills that you have acquired
- ☐ A chronology of your work experience that is easy to read
- ☐ Specialized training
- ☐ Certificates or licenses
- ☐ The title of each post you have held
- ☐ Details specific to each work experience
- ☐ Strong and varied verbs to highlight your strengths
- ☐ Professionalism, demonstrated through your format and language
- ☐ Skills delineated by jobs or categories
- ☐ Work dates
- ☐ Education and degrees
- ☐ Special skills, such as computer knowledge and second or third languages
- ☐ The language of the field used to articulate your skills

Thank-You Note

- ☐ Correct name of addressee and addresses
- ☐ Mention of the interview date and the position applied for
- ☐ Mention of the interview
- ☐ Your interest in position with that specific company
- ☐ A way to contact you
- ☐ A professional appearance of the note
- ☐ Professional language

UNIT PROOFREADING EXERCISES

Proofread the following letter and make the needed changes in grammar, spelling, and punctuation.

This letter of application is for the post of Licensed practical nurse that was advertised in The Chronicle on Sunday November 7 2004. The listing noted that the position required a respondsive and responsible individual to provide home health care needs to a retirement community. Having worked first as a home health care aide, I begin my health career by supporting my patients in the privacy of there own homes. I am licensed and trained in several areas that support issues such as end-of-life care, family counseling grieving and handling the wide variety of insurance paperwork. My luv for the elderly is what attracts me to the post.

UNIT REVISION EXERCISES

Read the following application to be a volunteer at a local hospital. Make any corrections necessary to ensure a professional and accurate application. Neatly add corrections to the application.

Meadowview Hospital Volunteer Application		
Name	Gretchen smith	
Address	23414 12th street West	
City, State, Zip	Los Angeles, CA 27654	
Home Phone	(213) 555-0100	
Work Phone		
Cell Phone	(753) 555-0199	
E-mail Address	smartgirl@yahoo.com	
Availability	☐ Weekday Mornings	☐ Weekday Mornings
	☐ Weekday Afternoons	☐ Weekday Afternoons
	☐ Weekday Evenings	☐ Weekday Evenings
	Other Specific Times ____________	
Available Start Date	___ Immediately ____________	
Interested Area for Volunteering	☒ Clerical Tasks	☐ Magazine Sorting
	☐ Customer Service	☐ Mail Delivery
	☐ Decorating Committee	☐ Phone Bank

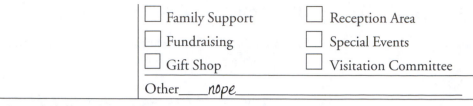

	☐ Family Support ☐ Reception Area ☐ Fundraising ☐ Special Events ☐ Gift Shop ☐ Visitation Committee
	Other nope
Special Skills and Qualifications	
Summarize special skills, qualifications, and attributes that you have gained through employment or previous volunteer work	
I am really fast typist and I like to do office work. Like filing, printing, mailing, and answerwering fones. I have recently retired. I need to so something.	
Summarize your previous volunteer experience	
I wanna get started giving back to the community. I have done charity work through my previous job and that inspires me to do more. I participate in "Senior walk-a-thong" for Alzhomiers research and "The Relay for Life" cancer benefit for the passed five years. I am active in my church.	
I affirm that the information in this application is true and complete.	
Signature/Date	GS

Was the previous volunteer application to volunteer complete and helpful to the person reviewing the application?

____

____

____

____

____

Rewrite the application below so that it is correct.

Meadowview Hospital Volunteer Application	
Name	Gretchen smith
Address	23414 12th street West
City, State, Zip	Los Angeles, CA 27654
Home Phone	(213) 555-0100
Work Phone	
Cell Phone	(753) 555-0199
E-mail Address	smartgirl@yahoo.com

Availability	☐ Weekday Mornings ☐ Weekday Afternoons ☐ Weekday Evenings Other Specific Times ____________	☐ Weekday Mornings ☐ Weekday Afternoons ☐ Weekday Evenings
Available Start Date		
Interested Area for Volunteering	☐ Clerical Tasks ☐ Customer Service ☐ Decorating Committee ☐ Family Support ☐ Fundraising ☐ Gift Shop Other____________	☐ Magazine Sorting ☐ Mail Delivery ☐ Phone Bank ☐ Reception Area ☐ Special Events ☐ Visitation Committee
Special Skills and Qualifications		
Summarize special skills, qualifications, and attributes that you have gained through employment or previous volunteer work		
Summarize your previous volunteer experience		
I affirm that the information in this application is true and complete.		
Signature/Date		

UNIT EXTENSIONS

1. Write your perfect job description. Be creative and don't forget to include the benefit package and retirement options you desire.
2. Write a letter to your instructor in which you discuss your progress in the course.
3. Critique your skills in a specific area. Use professional language and format.

UNIT 9 SELF-CHECK

1. What two important skills are used when writing summary sentences or paragraphs?
   a. ____________________
   b. ____________________

Revise each of the following job-related statements so that each appears professional and effective for applying for a job. Add content and improved language.

2. I wanna to be a certified nursing aid because my friends said it was a good job.

____

____

3. Thanks so much for considering my application.

____

____

4. I am really interested in this position.

____

____

5. This is the reason that I think this job is perfect for me.

____

____

6. Can you please call me for an interview?

____

____

Read the job application summary of Mr. Fred Peterson and revise the summary to clarify any ideas that would assist him in presenting himself to the prospective employer:

How can you tell us about yourself that might not be clear from your job application?

First of all, I do like all people. I wanna travel all over the world and meet people. I spoke Spanish. I participate in local health care charities. I got into the health care field as a nurses aid becus my aunt was old and needed a lot of care so I sort of started to help her out. Then I took a course and learned the skills I needed to work in a long-term care facility.

7. What are the apparent weaknesses presented in this summary?

____

____

Revision:

8. Write a summary paragraph form this table of information. The information is in no particular order.

What are head lice?	**What else should I do?**	**How are head lice spread?**
Lice are tiny insects that are gray, brown, or black. Lice crawl through hair. Lice lay eggs called nits on the hair shaft close to the scalp. Nits hatch in about 6 days. Nits are oval and attached to the hair shaft. They are easier than lice to spot.	*Check all members of the household. Treat all family members who have lice. Notify your child's school or daycare. Wash all combs, brushes, and hair clips in soapy water (above 129°F) for at least 10 minutes. Launder by washing and heat drying all clothing and bedding used by the infested person in the 48 hours before treatment for lice. Vacuum furniture and carpets and change the vacuum bag thereafter.*	*Anyone can become infested by head-to-head contact, by wearing another person's hat or using his or her comb or brush or bedding or by sharing clothing.*
How can lice outbreaks be prevented?	**How do I treat hair to get rid of lice?**	**What are symptoms of head lice?**
Check you child's hair weekly for lice or nits. Do not share combs, brushes, or clothing; store items separately at school; wash clothing and bedding.	*Lice and their eggs can be treated with Nix; follow package instructions exactly.*	*Itching of the scalp is the most common symptom.*
What if lice come back?	**Where can I get more information?**	**What is the medical name for head lice?**
You may reapply Nix again after 7–10 days; this is not usually necessary.	*Call your family doctor or public health department.*	*Pediculosis*

UNIT 10

Writing Skills with Process/Sequence

UNIT TERMS

Process	The series or steps from the beginning to the end of an action
Informative	Describes writing that explains how the steps come together or function together
Instructive	Describes writing that teaches through step-by-step instructions
Sequence	An order of first, second, third of a process or directions
Transition words	Words that join phrases and sentences

UNIT OBJECTIVES

Upon completion of this unit, the student should be able to

1. identify the paragraph as an instructive or informative process paragraph
2. write an instructive process paragraph
3. write an informative process paragraph
4. use effective transition words to join ideas and show the relationships between steps

Glossary of Medical Terms

Term	Part of Speech	Definition
anatomy	noun	the structure of an organism
diabetic	noun	one who has diabetes
fatigue	noun; verb	mental or physical exhaustion; to tire out
floss	noun; verb	a string used to clean between teeth; to clean
IV	noun	intravenous
physiology	noun	the science of the functions of living organisms and the parts
resistance	noun	the body's ability to remain unchanged by something
stress	noun	emotional, mental, or physical strain that affects the body

VOCABULARY OF PROCESS/SEQUENCE

Process paragraphs use words to help sequence the steps in a series. Sometimes, only the obvious words come to mind, such as *first*, *second*, *third*, and *finally*. Other options exist and can contribute to a paragraph's flow of information:

To Begin a Process	To Continue a Process	To End a Process
first	after	finally
begin with	as; as soon as	last
initially	before	the final step
to start	continue	to conclude
begin by	during	at last
in the first step	later	
	meanwhile	
	next	
	when	
	while	

Two types of process paragraphs exist, instructional and informative.

INSTRUCTIONAL PARAGRAPHS

An instructional process paragraph explains how something is done. The steps are laid out in sequence. These paragraphs are step-by-step instructions for a process.

INFORMATIONAL PARAGRAPHS

Informational process paragraphs explain how something was or is done with data and information to support why the process was done in that specific manner. These paragraphs are more analytical and explanatory than directional.

In healthcare, both types of process paragraphs exist. Instructional process paragraphs are used in training on equipment and new procedures, while informative process paragraphs are used with the explanations of the manifestation of health issues or the stages of a disease. Sometimes, a combination of forms occurs.

PROCESS/SEQUENTIAL PARAGRAPH

Normally, processes have multiple steps. Although there are specific processes that can be given in a sentence, the process paragraph is more common in healthcare. The process paragraph gives the reader step-by-step direction to complete a process or information about the process. In both cases, the key is that the steps are properly ordered, and the steps are easy to follow. If, as a writer, you find that a step is becoming too long and complicated, perhaps the process should be explained in multiple steps rather than a single step. Careful analysis of the process and its sequence will help you determine this.

The main-idea sentence will state clearly what the process is, what it is used for, and/or why it is important. The supporting paragraphs will actually provide the individual steps.

Time and the transition words usually order and help the reader follow the steps. Some time expressions are:

first	second	later
initially	afterward	before
begin by	then	as soon as
start with	next	finally
until	during	at last

Sometimes the steps will be enumerated, and then each step will be numbered, listed out, and separated. This assists the reader when a complex series of steps is required. The concluding sentence will provide a final step or a statement noting that the process is complete.

Process paragraphs are used frequently in healthcare to provide instructions in completing tasks. This style of writing is helpful as it orders and/or prioritizes the steps to be completed. When a family member is requesting information about caring for a patient, an instructive process paragraph can provide an effective format. Process paragraphs are most often used in instruction manuals and other guides that help consumers.

Think about the steps that you need to learn a new procedure:

> *Learning how to study for an anatomy and physiology test is the key to ensure successful course completion. First, purchase the required text and index cards. Second, plan and set aside your study time to ensure that the time is truly for dedicated study. Include time for unexpected emergencies, interruptions, and everyday happenings. Third, review the course outline carefully. Be sure of the point distributions, test dates, required readings, and other specific class details. Fourth, read the chapter once; wait a while and reread it. Underline the key definitions and write these on your index cards. Fifth, memorize the graphics and their labels. Later reread the chapter a third time and thereafter write the answers to the summary or review questions at the end of the chapter. Finally, collate class notes, your review questions, and the index cards with the terms on them and do a once-over, reviewing the graphics from the chapter, the notes, and the terminology. If you apply this technique for each chapter in anatomy and physiology course, you will be successfully prepared and stress free before exams.*

EXERCISE 10-1: Your texts have procedures, certain patient care routines, or equipment setup or sterilization techniques in them. Select one of these and read it several times. Then write down the steps in sequence. Not only will this help you learn the individual steps, but it will also help you memorize the order of the steps.

Exercise 10-2: Draft an *instructional* process paragraph on one of the following processes.

1. How to make a bed with a patient in it
2. How to set up a new IV
3. How to check a drug label for accuracy
4. How to provide superior customer service to your patients and their family members
5. How to (instructor-suggested topic)

Exercise 10-3: Draft an *informative* process paragraph on one of the following processes.

1. How a specific treatment plan is effective for helping diabetics or overweight patients manage their health
2. How medical research has provided new treatment options for certain cancers and diseases
3. How to gain a patient's trust about having an uncomfortable procedure
4. How the 12-step recovery process affects a person
5. How to (instructor's choice of topic)

Process/Sequence Paragraph Checklist

Check the appropriate box in response to each question.

☐ Yes ☐ No Is the process mentioned in the topic sentence?

☐ Yes ☐ No Are the steps provided in a logical way?

☐ Yes ☐ No Do the support sentences further define the distinguishing features?

☐ Yes ☐ No Do the support sentences show the sequence in the process effectively?

☐ Yes ☐ No Do transition words help unite the sentences and aid the reader in understanding the paragraph?

☐ Yes ☐ No Is there a concluding sentence?

☐ Yes ☐ No Does the concluding sentence draw the paragraph to a meaningful close?

☐ Yes ☐ No Has a spelling check been done?

☐ Yes ☐ No Are the sentences varied in length and content?

☐ Yes ☐ No Are the sentences punctuated correctly?

☐ Yes ☐ No Do subjects and verbs agree?

USING PROCESS TO LEARN MEDICAL PROCEDURES

In science and technology, students read a wide variety of process paragraphs and essays. One technique that comes from these industries is the task-flow diagram. It can be very helpful in drafting information for planning a process paragraph or educating a patient about a sequence of steps:

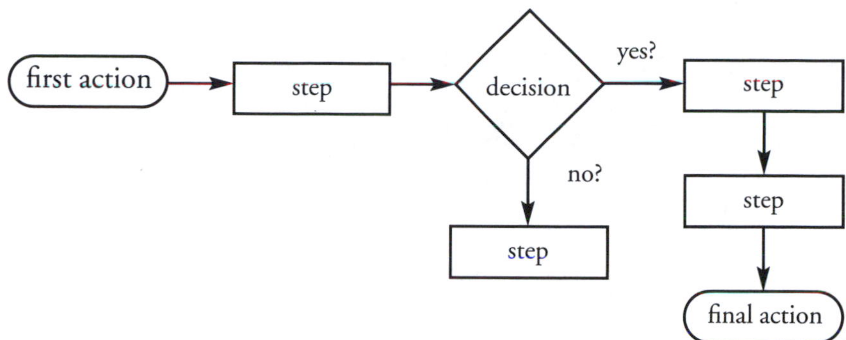

Although there are many symbols used for developing a task-flow diagram, the basics are as shown below.

Symbol	Purpose in a Task-Flow Diagram
(rounded rectangle)	Shows the first and the final steps
(rectangle)	Used for each of the steps in a series
(diamond)	Represents a decision-making box; usually has two offshoots, a *yes* and a set of steps that correspond to it and a *no* and a set of the steps that follow that line of reasoning
(arrow)	Shows the direction of the steps or actions to be sequenced

Task-flow diagrams help writers organize their thoughts by illustrating a process. These diagrams can be simple or complex.

Preparing for an exam

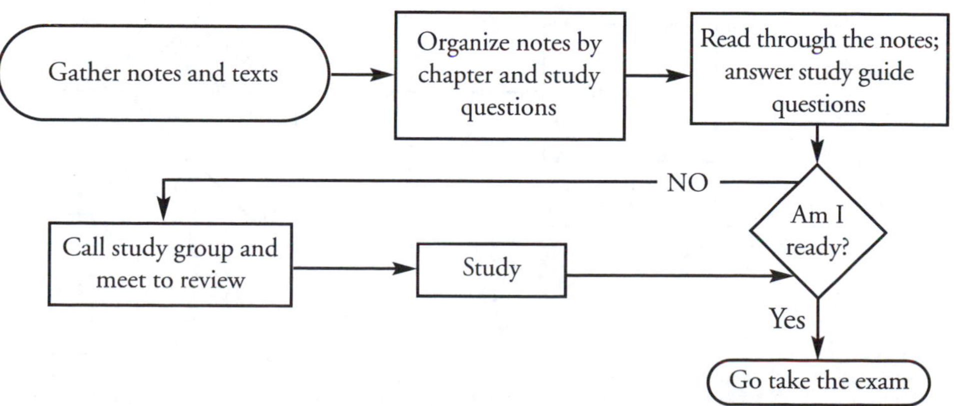

EXERCISE 10-4: Think about a task that you will do or are learning how to do to be a healthcare professional. Illustrate it in a task-flow diagram.

UNIT PROOFREADING EXERCISES

Compare the task-flow diagram with the paragraph below it. Assume that the task-flow diagram is the accurate information. Circle the inconsistencies in the paragraph. Then rewrite the paragraph so that it accurately describes the task-flow diagram.

Step-by-Step Flossing

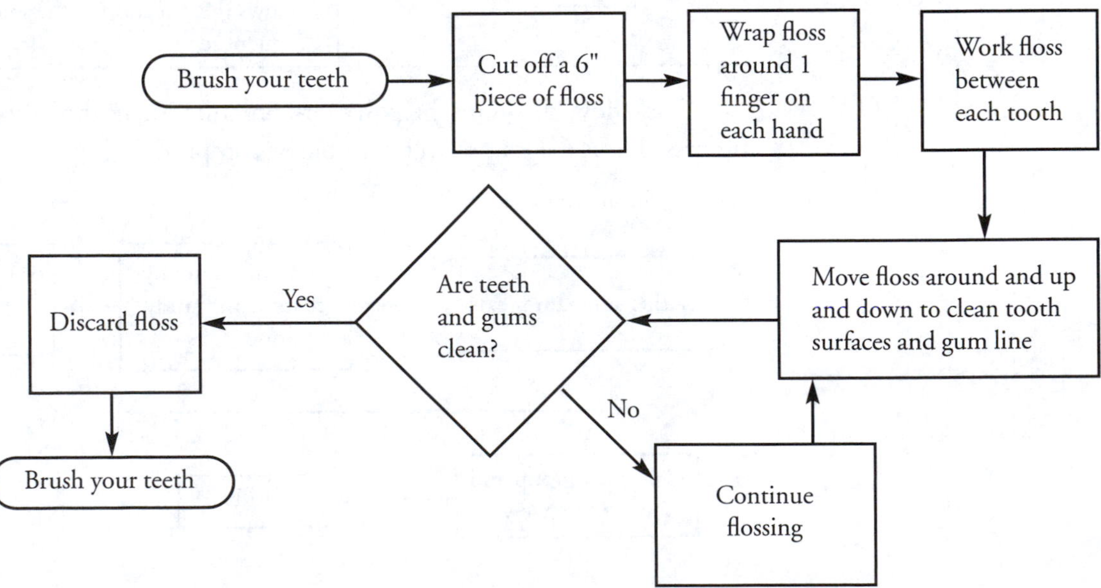

Step-by-Step Flossing

> *First brush your teeth. Wrap a piece of floss between two fingers. The floss should be cut into a six-inch piece. Push floss down, around, and back and forth between the teeth. Continue flossing. If the gum is cleaned, brush teeth. Discard floss.*

Revision:

____

____

____

____

____

____

____

____

UNIT REVISION EXERCISES

Read the following paragraph and make the following changes. First, reorder sentences that may be out of order. Then, add transition words to add clarity between the steps.

> Stress must be managed. One definition of stress is a human being's response to physical, intellectual, or emotional pressures. If stress is endured for long periods of time, the human body uses its defenses, and it will enter a stage of exhaustion or extreme fatigue. Stress has three fundamental stages: alarm, resistance, and exhaustion. Another definition is the mind's and body's reaction to either imagined or real threats, events, or situations. A situation is defined as stressful by our perception of the stimulus creating the stress. The body's first reaction to stress is a physical reaction called fight-or-flight. There is a sudden release of the hormones epinephrine and norepinephrine. This hormone release increases the blood flow to the muscles, which, in turn, improves muscle strength and mental ability. Another state is called resistance. The body begins to cope by adapting to the stress, and this appears to build resistance to the stress. In other words, your body handles the stress better. Stress is an internal reaction to the events that all people encounter; what matters is how we respond to it.

____

____

____

____

UNIT EXTENSIONS

1. Write a paragraph describing a common process you do on the job.
2. Draw a task-flow diagram for a routine task in patient care.
3. Look at an over-the-counter skin-care product and draft a process paragraph detailing the instructions.

UNIT 10 SELF-CHECK

1. Read the following sentences; then arrange them in sequential order.

______ **a.** Place the thermometer in the healthcare facility's chemical solution for the prescribed time or in 90% alcohol.

______ **b.** Dry the thermometer after rinsing it with water.

______ **c.** Clean the thermometer with soap or detergent solution, rubbing it with firm strokes.

______ **d.** Use a soft, clean tissue or gauze to wipe the thermometer.

______ **e.** Rinse the thermometer under cold running water.

______ **f.** Rinse the thermometer in warm water after disinfecting it and store in a dry place.

______ **g.** Hold the tissue or gauze at the thermometer's stem and wipe downward toward the bulb. Twist firmly as you wipe downward.

2. Select a process you will do as a healthcare professional. It can be something such as changing a colostomy bag or calculating a medication dosage. List the steps in sequential order from start to finish. Then draft a paragraph describing this process.

UNIT 11

Writing Skills with Analysis

UNIT TERMS

Analysis	An examination of the parts of a whole to determine the role each part plays in creating the whole
Parts of speech	Nouns, verbs, adjectives, adverbs, prepositions, conjunctions, interjections, pronouns

UNIT OBJECTIVES

Upon completion of this unit, the student will be able to

1. define analysis
2. use analysis to assist in fill-in-the-blank type questions
3. draft an analytical paragraph

Glossary of Medical Terms

Term	Part of Speech	Definition
asthma	noun	a respiratory disease characterized by coughing and breathing difficulties
bile	noun	yellow-green fluid produced by the liver; fluid used in digestion to emulsify fats
clinical	adjective	based on medical treatment, diagnosis, and observation
cryosurgery	noun	a surgical technique that exposes tissue to extreme cold
endoscopy	noun	an internal examination by the endoscope
impetigo	noun	an inflammatory skin disease that has skin pustules
inflammatory	adjective	becoming inflamed in response to injury or disease
irreversible	adjective	cannot be reversed; unable to undo
jaundice	noun	a condition of excess bilirubin in the blood; characterized by yellowing skin, whites of the eyes, and mucous membranes
macrophage	noun	a monocyte that has settled into the alveoli, spleen, tonsils, or lymph nodes
necrosis	noun	death of tissue
nephrons	noun	the structural and functional parts of the kidney
nodular	adjective	like a node or lump or cluster of cells
oncologist	noun	a specialist in tumors
pathologist	noun	a specialist in diagnosing changes in tissue samples
pavor nocturnus	noun	an anxiety disorder or condition that creates frightening night terrors

posttraumatic stress disorder	noun	a set of symptoms that develop after psychological trauma
prostate	noun	a gland that surrounds the neck of the bladder and the urethra in males
swelling	noun	an abnormal enlargement of an area
therapist	noun	a person skilled in giving therapy
urologist	noun	a physician specializing in the urinary tract
viscera	noun	internal organs that are enclosed in a cavity
wheezing	noun	the whistling sound produced during difficult breathing

USING LANGUAGE ANALYSIS IN THE WORKPLACE

Analysis is used to evaluate a process, problems, or situations. We use analysis every day when we make decisions. Test questions, procedures, flowcharts, manuals, and patients' care charts are all examples of situations in which we see and use analytical writing.

Our workplace represents people of diverse backgrounds. Our choice of language is central to respecting others and to our being professionals. Language speaks of our level of education; therefore, an individual who analyzes his or her language may use different words and phrases. Use specific and clear language. For example:

He was <u>sort of</u> frustrated at me.
He was frustrated at me for being careless with my documentation.

Carefully think through the words you use to ensure clear communication. This is especially true for documenting accidents, problems, and incidents between staff and patients. Look at the following example:

Incident of April 2, 2007
I was just workin and I noticed Bob staring at me. Then he whispered something to Fred. I got mad becuz they always be talking and goofin off when de boss is in a meeting and I am doing all the work. It's notfair so I yelled at those dudes, but latter I told em I was sorry.

Exercise 11-1: List the facts and opinions in the incident report of April 2, 2007, above.

Incident Report: April 2, 2007	
Facts	**Opinions**

By reviewing the table above, it is clear that there are as many opinions as facts in the incident report. The report is an emotional response to a situation that upset an individual. Now read the following revised memo:

Incident of April 2, 2007

On Monday April 2, 2007, at 9:30 a.m., I was making patient beds in Wing C on the second floor. I was distracted by the whispering of Bob Maestro and Fred Johnson who appeared to be making fun of me. I knew that Mr. Brown was in a meeting, and I could not leave my work area to locate the Head Nurse. I raised my voice at them to try to let them know that I did not appreciate their behavior. That was a poor choice of actions on my part. I immediately apologized to Fred and the patients and staff in the hallway.

EXERCISE 11-2: List the facts and opinions in the incident report of April 2, 2007, above.

Incident Report: April 2, 2007	
Facts	**Opinions**

By reviewing the table above, it is clear that there are more facts than opinions in the incident report. The report is a professional response to a situation that an individual found himself in during the course of his day. Notice that the language has been elevated to professional terms.

EXERCISE 11-3: Revise the following memos, notes, and incident reports. You may add any details to clarify and improve the communication.

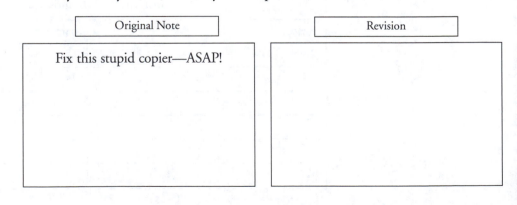

Original Note	Revision
Fix this stupid copier—ASAP!	

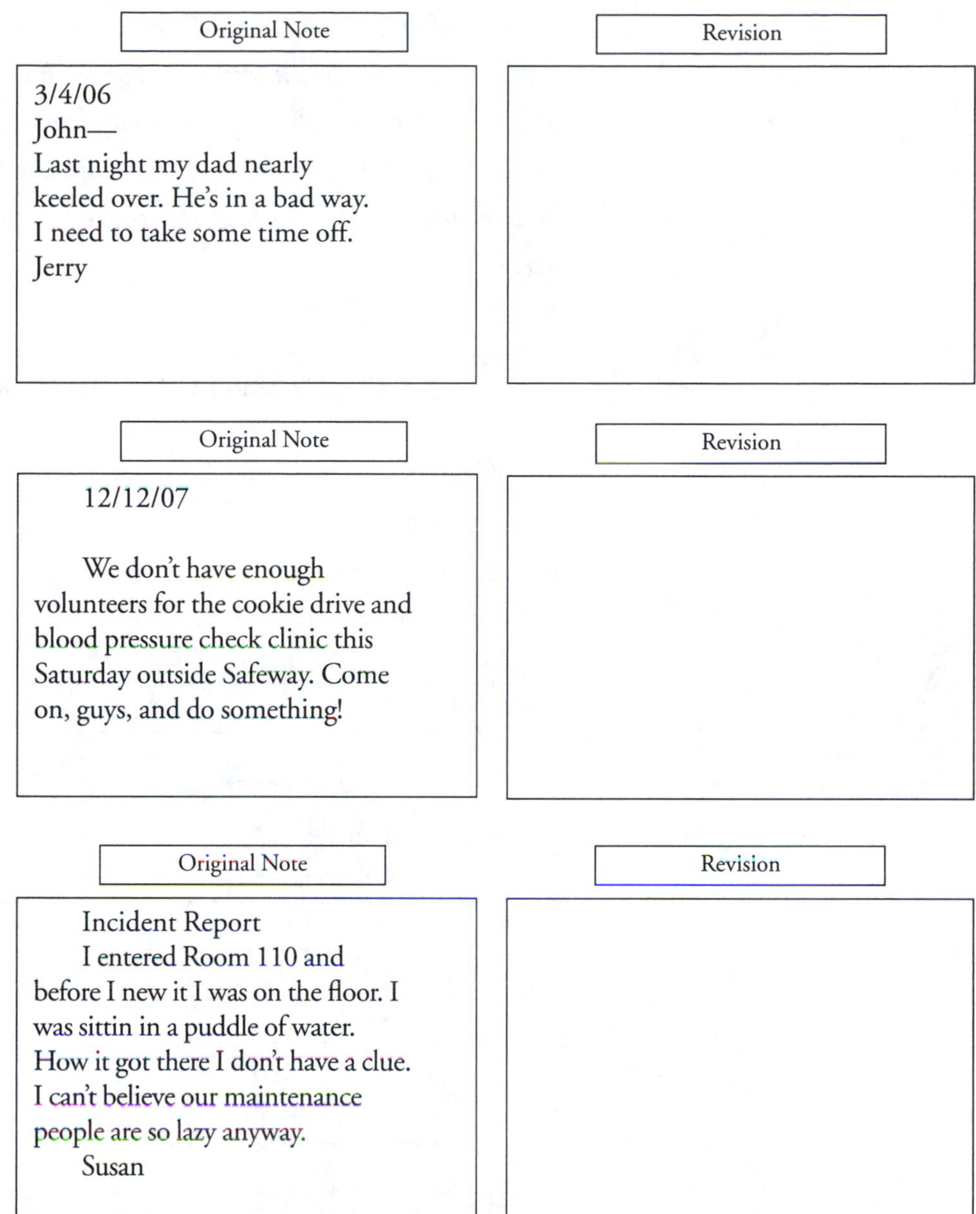

Original Note	Revision
3/4/06 John— Last night my dad nearly keeled over. He's in a bad way. I need to take some time off. Jerry	

Original Note	Revision
12/12/07 We don't have enough volunteers for the cookie drive and blood pressure check clinic this Saturday outside Safeway. Come on, guys, and do something!	

Original Note	Revision
Incident Report I entered Room 110 and before I new it I was on the floor. I was sittin in a puddle of water. How it got there I don't have a clue. I can't believe our maintenance people are so lazy anyway. Susan	

Workplaces all have their own incident or accident forms that employees are expected to fill out if they are involved in an incident. These forms are necessary to document accidents and injuries in the workplace. Accuracy and specifics are necessary to complete these forms.

EXERCISE 11-4: Read the situation below and then complete the incident form, adding information to complete each line. For example, you will need to provide a name and address on this incident form.

On Saturday afternoon at 12:25, I was delivering a hot food tray to Mrs. Brown in room 234. As I turned into room 234, a visitor, Frieda Berkshure, was exiting the room. I did not see Ms. Berkshure coming out of the room, and I ran into her, spilling the tray and upsetting Mrs. Brown. The dishes dropped off the tray, and hot water sprayed everywhere. No hot water hit Frieda Berkshure or Mrs. Brown. As I picked up the broken glass, I cut my hand across the palm. I immediately applied pressure. I called a nurse to assist me. I went to the doctor immediately and had fifteen stitches put in my right hand. I returned to work and told Mr. Smith what happened. He told me to take the rest of the day off.

CITY HOSPITAL INCIDENT REPORT

Name of individual(s) involved: ______________________

Place of incident: ______________________

Date and time of incident: ______________________

Incident was reported to:

____

____

____

Description of the incident:

____

____

____

____

____

____

____

____

____

____

____

____

Follow-up action needed:

____

____

____

____

Report submitted by: ____________________ Date of report: __________

EXERCISE 11-5: Read the situation below and then complete the incident form, adding information to complete each line. For example, you will need to provide a name and address on this incident form.

> *I was driving the company vehicle to pick up some office supplies from Office Central. When I returned to the lot, I did not see that the garbage dumpster had been moved. I hit the edge of the dumpster with the right fender of the vehicle. I dented the fender. There is a 9-inch dent in the fender of the car. I was not hurt. The dumpster did not get damaged. The fender has the dent plus some paint was scraped off in the process. My insurance company is Allstate and my policy number is TR-45783-234. I was on duty when this accident occurred. I reported this accident to my supervisor, Bob Gregory, and to the head of maintenance, who handled the Pacific Rim Care and Reh. Center's vehicle. I had no witnesses.*

PACIFIC RIM CARE AND REHABILITATION CENTER
ACCIDENT AND INCIDENT REPORT

Please print in black ink

Personal Information

Full Name of Injured Person

☐ Employee ☐ Visitor ☐ Trainee ☐ Public ☐ Contractor ☐ Other

Address:

Job Title:	Date of Birth:
Work Phone:	Home Phone:

Accident/Incident Details

☐ Accidental Injury ☐ Threatening Behavior/Verbal ☐ Physical Violence ☐ Other (Specify):

Date: Time: Documentation ☐ yes ☐ no

Witnesses:

What was the injured person doing at the time of accident?

If employee, how long in this position?

Who was in charge?

Were others involved? ☐ yes ☐ no If yes, specify:

Was equipment involved? ☐ yes ☐ no If yes, specify:

(continued)

Accident/Incident Details Continued	
Were there injuries ☐ yes ☐ no If yes, specify:	
Were the injuries treated by a medical professional? ☐ yes ☐ no If yes, specify treatment:	
For employees:	
If absence from work expected, specify in days:	
This information is correct and true as stated:	
Signature:	Date:

USING GRAMMAR KNOWLEDGE TO ANALYZE FILL-IN-THE-BLANK QUESTIONS

Analysis allows us to make educated guesses for fill-in-the-blank test questions. If we look at the structure and words in a fill-in-the-blank sentence, we are able to gain clues about what must be filled in by relying on analysis. This analysis requires that we rely on our basic knowledge of English sentence structure.

Recall a few basic rules:

1. The articles, *a/an/the*, are followed by a noun. There may be an adjective before the noun, but ultimately there must be a noun in this word group. For example:

   A __________ met with the doctor. (patient, therapist, counselor, relative)

   An __________ is the specialist that I am referring you to for a consultation. (oncologist, urologist)

   The __________ felt he needed help. (patient, therapist, counselor, relative)

2. An article is often followed by an adjective, then a noun. So if a term comes between the article and the noun, most likely it will be an adjective:

   a __________ finding (clinical, research, scientific)

   a __________ position (clinical, research, scientific)

   the __________ condition (pathological, irreversible)

3. Usually a noun is followed by a verb:

   the nasal passage __________ (blocked, damaged, remains)

   the union __________ (negotiated, bargains, reversed)

4. A gerund (verb + *ing*) functions as a noun. These are generally used as subjects in sentences, and they describe an activity. Gerunds are singular subjects. A gerund or gerund phrase as subject is followed by a singular verb:

__________ the cause of the disease is critical.

Establishing the cause of the disease is critical.

__________ is important to the foundation.

Generating funds is important to the foundation.

__________ the sites is our best option.

Incising the sites is our best option.

5. Prepositional phrases begin with a preposition and end in a noun or pronoun:

in __________ (examining) = in examining

of __________ (scrape) = of scraping

by __________ (doctor) = by the doctor

Exercise 11-6: Choose words from the chart below to complete the paragraph.

condition	yellow	symptoms	icterus
enters	bile	yellowing	jaundice

One of the __________ of liver disease or problems is the __________ of the skin. __________ is the name of the condition when the skin turns __________. This __________ is also known as __________.

A __________ duct may be blocked. In this case, the bile __________ the bloodstream.

Knowing the parts of speech is a benefit because it will ensure that on fill-in-the-blank tests you are able to use the correct form of the word. This means that your answer will be accurate. For example:

The endoscopy procedure took thirty-five minutes. (Incorrect: Endoscopy is a noun; in this situation, the adjective form of the word is required to be grammatically correct.)

The endoscopic procedure took thirty-five minutes. (Correct: adjective form used.)

Exercise 11-7: Use the words in the chart below to complete the fill-in-the-blank statements. The word should be consistent with medical use of the term and fit the context.

efficiently	procedure
in the room	immediately
warm	in turmoil
scraped	diet
will exhaust	dental

1. The ____________________ (*noun*) was performed by the technician.
2. The ____________________ (*adjective*) procedure made the patient feel nervous.
3. The dental assistant ____________________ (*action verb*) the tartar from the bicuspid.
4. Meeting the family ____________________ (*prepositional phrase*), the head nurse ensured they were apprised of the patient's progress.
5. The surgical technologist returned to the surgery suite ____________________ (*adverb*).
6. The energy needed to breathe ____________________ (*verb phrase*) an ill person.
7. ____________________ (*prepositional phrase*), the staff cannot function efficiently.
8. The procedure was completed ____________________ (*adverb*).
9. By watching your ____________________ (*noun*), you will lose weight.
10. ____________________ (*adjective*) baths may help the patient feel more comfortable.

ANALYTICAL PARAGRAPHS

Analytical paragraphs require careful thought and development so that the reader is given creditable information from which to base a decision or form an opinion. For this reason, an analytical paragraph needs to have certain types of information:

1. The information must be complete. Partial or incomplete data may be erroneous or one sided.
2. Information should be objective, scientific, and proven or provable. Biased data is unethical.
3. Information needs to be verifiable. Use facts and figures that can be substantiated.
4. Information needs to be specific. General information usually does not allow a reader to make an unbiased decision.

An analytical paragraph or report will feature the discrete parts that are critical to the specific topic being discussed. An analytical piece of writing may be an evaluation of a specific surgical technique, a choice of one medication over another, a review of treatment, an assessment of behavior and results of therapy. Another type of analysis is a self-evaluation, which most students have had an opportunity to do. When two items are being evaluated, the same features or characteristics need to be analyzed. Note that sometimes terms must be defined or at least placed in the correct context. In addition, an analytical paragraph often ends in a recommendation or suggestion, which follows logically from the data and information presented:

I consider myself a healthy person; however, I have noticed that my exercise regime is not doing the task I set out to accomplish: to lose weight and keep it off. My exercise regime included walking between five and seven miles a day. This plan was initially coupled with my drinking between 64 and 80 ounces of water each day. The reason that my weight has begun to slowly edge up the scale again is two-fold. I have reduced my mileage to approximately two miles a day, and sometimes I skip a day for various reasons. Next, I have literally stopped drinking water over the winter months. In addition, my food intake has increased. To resume weight loss, I need to resume my fluid intake and walk each day and for at least six miles per day at approximately 4.3 miles per hour; furthermore, I must avoid excessive sweets by exchanging them for a piece of fresh fruit. In doing so, I will once again gain control of my weight and as a result have more energy and look and feel better.

Another example of an analysis paragraph follows:

It is becoming increasingly more difficult for teens to maintain healthy lifestyles. Practicing healthy diet habits and being physically fit are often placed as last priorities by today's teens. Eating healthily has become an inconvenience and a hassle. Healthy foods often have to be searched for, whereas unhealthy foods are to be found anywhere. Healthy foods are becoming less common, and fatty foods are thriving in restaurants. Tasty junk foods and sugar-loaded pop are widely available in school vending machines while the plain, dull salad is often the only healthy food schools offer. Even if a teen chose to eat healthily, it often would cost more than eating fatty foods. The prices of the new carb-cutter trend meals are bumped up absurdly higher than the prices of greasy foods. Most teens, especially college students, do not have this extra change to spare for three meals a day, three-hundred and sixty-five days a year. Exercise has also become a neglected practice in teen life. It is a time-consuming, regular practice that most teens do not have the time for. High school often brings the burden of homework, and life often brings the burden of a part-time job. Teens need their education, and teens need their money. They view education and employment as influences on their futures that have more significance than exercise, and therefore exercise is pushed to the bottom of the priority pyramid. A health-conscious lifestyle is considered the ideal lifestyle for any individual, but oftentimes it is not a reality among teens.

Written by Robert Do, high school student, 3/25/2005

EXERCISE 11-8: Draft an analytical paragraph on *one* of the following topics:

1. Review the food pyramid at www.mypyramid.gov. Track your diet for seven days. Compare your diet for a week with the recommendations

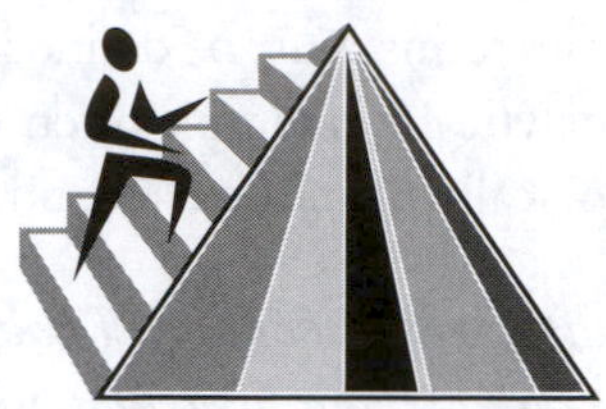

Graphic by U.S. Department of Agriculture and the U.S. Department of Health and Human Services

of the food pyramid. Provide an analysis of your diet and then develop a plan for reaching the suggested daily servings of the food pyramid. Note the changes or adjustments that need to be made to your diet.

2. Review Maslow's theory and analyze the needs of the elderly in a residential care facility according to this hierarchy of needs. Cite specifics.
3. Review Erickson's theory and analyze the needs of children in day care.
4. Consider lifestyle choices that promote a lifetime of health. Draft a self-analysis of your lifestyle and the improvements you can make to improve the quality of life and your healthiness.
5. Patients of all types have certain healthcare expectations. Analyze the key expectations that patients have of healthcare providers and then self-analyze your role as a healthcare professional. Are you meeting the expectations of your patients?

Analysis Paragraph Checklist

Check the appropriate box in response to each question:

☐ Yes ☐ No Is the subject to be analyzed mentioned in the topic sentence?

☐ Yes ☐ No Do the support sentences further analyze the subject?

☐ Yes ☐ No Are the support sentences adequate to provide a complete analysis?

☐ Yes ☐ No Do transition words help unite the sentences and aid the reader in understanding the paragraph?

☐ Yes ☐ No Is there a concluding sentence?

☐ Yes ☐ No Does the concluding sentence draw the paragraph to a meaningful close?

☐ Yes ☐ No Has a spelling check been done?

☐ Yes ☐ No Are the sentences varied in length and content?

☐ Yes ☐ No Are the sentences punctuated correctly?

☐ Yes ☐ No Do subjects and verbs agree?

UNIT PROOFREADING EXERCISES

Read the following paragraph. There are five errors in word use. Locate them and make the corrections:

> Leishmania is a parasite disease of the skin, viscera, or mucous membrous. Leishmaniasis is caused by leishmania, which is transmitted to people via the bite of infected female sand flies. Leishmania organisms infect and reproduction in the macrophages. These organisms are controlled by a T-cell mediated response. Leshmania cutaneous is a chronic ulerationing, nodular skin lesion prevalent in tropical regions. Treatment options are somewhat limited and available only throught the Centers for Disease Control by a doctor.

UNIT REVISION EXERCISES

Revise the sentences to ensure the correct use of the terms. You may find using a medical dictionary to be helpful. Each sentence has one error that is underlined. Write the correction on the line provided.

1. Integumentarial is derived from the Latin term for covering.

   ____

2. He is scheduled for an endoscopy examination.

   ____

3. Under a microscope, kidney tissue revealed approximately 1 million nephrons filtering units. ______________________________

4. Necrotis is the death of cells, tissues, or organs.

   ____

5. Assessing the posttrauma stress patients requires a lot of documentation.

   ____

6. A phlebography or venography is a radiographic of the veins to identify and locate abnormalities in the veins of the lower extremities.

   ____

7. Impetigo is an inflame skin disease that is marked by pustules that become crusty and rupture. ______________________________

8. Selecting a prime care physician from all the available family medicine doctors is a challenge. ______________________________

9. Pavor nocturnus is a condition of anxious of the young or aged; it occurs during the night and is known as "night terrors."

   ____

10. Excising prostate tumors is one of the new cryosurgical that Dr. Wills has perfected. ______________________

UNIT EXTENSIONS

1. Purchase three different snack foods from the same category of food (three different types of chips, three different candy bars, three different fruit bars, or the like.) Compare the information on the labels. Develop a chart that compares the products in nutritional values, calories, flavor, texture, and so on. Write an analytical paragraph with the information that you have learned about the snacks.
2. Analyze your strongest professional attribute or skill. In a paragraph, provide the details about this attribute or skill and explain its benefit to the professional environment of the workplace.
3. Do an analysis of your local or regional job market for the health field. Use the Internet to search the state government growth predictions for the field. Draft a paragraph with the results.

UNIT 11 SELF-CHECK

1. Use the words below to fill in the blanks:

air	wheezing	asthma	reach
increase	constriction	illness	airways
SOB	hospitalization	severe	inflammatory

Asthma is an ______________ respiratory ______________, which is characterized by mild to ______________ difficulty in breathing. ______________ and swelling of the ______________ and an ______________ in mucous secretion close the smaller passages. When this occurs, ______________ cannot ______________ the lungs. ______________ occurs as the air is forced through the narrowed passage. An ______________ attack can create shortness of breath (______________) and may lead to ______________ .

2. Fill in the parts of speech. Put an *X* in a box if a form of the term does not exist.

Noun	Verb	Adjective
medicine		
		allergic
	excise	
diagnosis		
		idiopathic

3. Write an analytical paragraph. Use a health-related topic from your personal life or one social issue that interests you. Keep an objective point of view.

UNIT 12

Writing an Essay

UNIT TERMS

Annotated bibliography	A reference citation and an evaluative description of the material
APA	American Psychological Association
Body paragraph	Paragraph that supports the thesis with examples, details, and evidence
Concluding paragraph	Paragraph at the end of the essay that draws the essay to a close
Introductory paragraph	The first paragraph, which sets the tone of the paper and includes the thesis of the essay
MLA	Modern Language Association
Paraphrase	To use your own words to restate someone else's written or spoken work
Thesis statement	The controlling idea or argument of the essay written in one sentence
Topic	The subject of the writing
Transitions	Words, phrases, or clauses that connect related ideas to form a consistent argument or point of view

UNIT OBJECTIVES

Upon completion of this unit, the student should be able to

1. list the parts an essay
2. write an effective thesis statement
3. draft an introductory paragraph
4. draft support paragraphs
5. draft a concluding paragraph
6. write an annotated bibliography in APA format
7. use in-text citations properly

Glossary of Medical Terms

Term	Part of Speech	Definition
epidemic	noun	a disease that spreads quickly through a group of people
hospice	noun	home care for the dying or terminally ill
obesity	noun	the condition of being overweight or weighing more than 20% above the recommended weight for one's age and height
prenatal	adjective	before childbirth
supplement	noun	a food substance with a particular food value

THESIS STATEMENT

A thesis statement is a sentence that controls the content of a paper and expresses the writer's attitude about a subject. An effective thesis statement will include these four attributes:

1. expresses a main idea in specific terms
2. asserts a point or conclusion about a subject
3. deals with the subject matter in a way that meets the assignment
4. uses specific or limiting language

Thesis statements help writers in several ways. A thesis statement helps a writer put his or her argument in words that are specific and pointed. A thesis statement helps a writer organize and plan a composition. A thesis statement helps guide the reader through the paper.

What makes a strong thesis statement?

- An effective thesis statement is specific, and it tells the reader exactly what the paper will cover. The thesis must be able to be adequately covered within the composition; in other words, too general a topic is too hard to write about in a specific page count.

  Prenatal care is very important. *(weak thesis statement)*

  Prenatal care can detect conditions early and ensure adequate parent education prior to the birth of the baby. *(improved thesis statement)*

- An effective thesis statement expresses one main idea or one main point.

  Prenatal care is good. *(weak thesis statement)*

  Prenatal care is in the best interests of the mother and child's health. *(improved thesis statement)*

- An effective thesis statement will promote thinking and maybe even debate.

  Prenatal care should be a given. *(weak thesis statement)*

  Prenatal care should begin prior to a planned pregnancy, be covered for all women, and include genetic, nutrition, and fitness counseling. *(improved thesis statement)*

Many effective thesis statements show how ideas are related. This might appear in a nursing assignment that asks that two medical journal articles be compared or contrasted. Many clear and effective thesis statements include words like *because, so, so that, unless, however,* and *although*. These words help show the relationships betweens phrases and ideas. Furthermore, such terms can help narrow the topic to be more specific and manageable.

If the essay is an open topic, one way to decide what to write about is to ask questions about the topic. Once a writer settles on a question that is to be developed, he or she will make assertions to draft the thesis statement. In courses for college, oftentimes the topics are given, and a writer can use a formulaic means for beginning to develop a thesis. Then, as a writer becomes more confident, the style and details of the thesis statement may be embellished.

USING THE TOPIC TO LEAD INTO DEVELOPING AN EFFECTIVE THESIS STATEMENT

Most essay topics come in two parts, the background information and the question, which is the argument you are putting forth. Essays usually express a writer's opinion or summarize research in response to a question.

Do *not* think of the background information as the question. The purpose of the background information is to provide ideas about the topic, assist the writer in using appropriate words, and get the writer thinking about asserting a point about the subject matter.

EXERCISE 12-1: Look at the topic and essay question below. Circle the background information. Then, underline the question. Box any key words that could be used in an effective thesis statement in response to this assignment.

> Healthcare offers individuals a wide variety of career options and ladders for professional growth. Many people decide on the healthcare field because they like to help others. Others have experienced good quality of care in the field and want to contribute to the profession. How did you decide upon the specific field you chose in healthcare? Write a composition in which you detail your choice, how you made the decision, and why. Be specific and use examples to support your views.

Look at the examples of thesis statements below:

To become a nurse is my educational goal *because* the field is rapidly expanding, nurses provide an important service, *and* I can touch the lives of many individuals.

Choosing a career in nursing was easy *because* I have many role models who are in the profession, *and* the career options for nurses are varied, *and* there is a high demand for nurses.

Medical assistant is my career choice because this field combines office skills *and* patient care; both of these skills are present in my work experience.

Studying surgical technology allows me to use my organizational skills *and* offers me a career using the latest technology within the health professions.

Notice that a thesis can be developed in this format: Lead-in information from the essay topic's question + the word *because* or *by* + reason 1, reason 2, and reason 3.

Writers can use this format to draft a preliminary thesis statement, and this format will save writers time in trying to decide how to draft a thesis.

EXERCISE 12-2: Read the following essay topics. Draft a thesis statement for these topics. Use the words in the question as a lead-in for your answer. Make sure that your answer has a *because* and *two or three specific reasons for your opinion or argument.*

Topic 1: Over the past few years, many people are making the connection between diet and health. We have more grocery stores than ever before. People are watching cooking shows on television and discussing about their meals like never before.

In a composition, state what you believe that connection is and what impact that has on you. Give specific examples to support your view.

Thesis Statement:

____

____

____

Topic 2: Some communities offer excellent community health programs that serve those who have limited access or limited resources to medicine and healthcare. Visiting nurses, hospices, and community clinics help fill the gap and provide services that are also available from formal healthcare settings.

Write a composition discussing the role of the public health department in providing equable services to the community at large. Be sure to include specific examples to support your views.

Thesis Statement:

____

____

____

Topic 3: Americans spend billions of dollars on their vitamins, supplements, and medications. Some of these are over-the-counter products, while others are prescribed.

In a composition, explain why you think vitamins, supplements, and medications are so important to people. Be specific and use examples to support your reasons.

Thesis Statement:

____

____

____

Topic 4: What are the advantages of shopping for your medications out of the country? Some people drive to Canada or Mexico. The largest reason for individuals doing this is the lower price offered for the same products.

Write a composition of about 200 words that discusses the advantages of buying medications abroad. Be sure to include specific examples to support your views.

Thesis Statement:

____

____

____

Topic 5: Today, computers are part of our lives. Hospitals, clinics, medical laboratories, and doctor's offices rely on advanced technologies to diagnose, monitor, and document patients' healthcare information.

Write a composition that discusses the role of technology and its effect on the healthcare industry. You may wish to deal with the good effects, bad effects, or both. Be sure to be specific and use examples to support your views.

Thesis Statement:

____

____

____

WHAT DOES A COMPOSITION LOOK LIKE?

An essay or composition is a compilation of several different paragraphs:

Introductory Paragraph

- introduces the topic
- establishes a point of reference
- ends with the thesis statement

Body Paragraphs

- evidence
- support
- examples

Concluding Paragraph

- draws the essay to a close
- does not introduce new concepts
- lets the reader know that the essay is complete

WRITING THE FIRST PARAGRAPH

The first paragraph is the most important paragraph in the entire essay.

The first paragraph should

1. introduce the topic
2. provide a context for the reader
3. warm the reader to the subject
4. respond to the topic or question with two or three specific reasons (thesis statement)

To accomplish these, it is important that you plan your introductory paragraph.

Indent the first paragraph. Write three sentences that introduce the topic to the reader. These sentences can be simple and straightforward.

No specific details or examples should be given in the first paragraph. The final sentence of the paragraph is the thesis that answers the question. It should include *the lead-in* and the word *because* followed by *two specific reasons.*

> Food, cooking, and shopping opportunities meet us around every street corner and shopping aisle. We are a society of consumers, food-wise and money-wise. Television shows and glossy magazine covers encourage cooking and eating. Overeating has become an epidemic because Americans have lost their desire to consume healthy foods in limited portions, and the majority of Americans have a weight problem.

Answer to the question (thesis statement)

EXERCISE 12-3: Choose one of the thesis statements that you developed from the previous pages. Draft an introductory paragraph. Remember that the thesis statement should be the final sentence in the introductory paragraph. Indent the first line.

____

____

____

____

____

____

____

____

____

____

WRITING SUPPORT PARAGRAPHS

What does a support paragraph look like? Each support paragraph begins with a topic sentence, which restates the point from your thesis. Next are the details and examples for your opinion. Finally, a concluding sentence ends the paragraph.

Support paragraphs provide the ideas, examples, and details that support your main-idea sentence. This is the place to explain what you know or feel about the topic.

Support paragraphs provide a lot of different kinds of information:

- researched information
- data and facts
- examples from your personal life
- information you have read
- an analogy showing your point
- personal experience relevant to the topic

Look at the thesis statement from the example paragraph:

Overeating has become an epidemic because Americans have lost their desire to consume healthy foods in limited portions, *(Reason 1)* and the majority of Americans have a weight problem. *(Reason 2)*

Use the first reason to write the topic sentence of the first support paragraph:

first topic sentence

Americans no longer limit their intake to nutritional needs; instead, Americans buy or order more food than they can or should eat. Portions have been doubled or tripled by biggy fries and supersized meals. In addition to this, we eat fiberless, fatty foods that offer diminished food value. Often the meals are eaten on the run, in our cars, or at our desks, so there is no sense of consumption durations or quantities. Thus, Americans consume excessive amounts of food, yet still find themselves hungering for another bite.

The second reason in the example thesis is

Overeating has become an epidemic because . . . the majority of Americans have a weight problem. *(Reason 2)*

second topic sentence

Overeating in America has created an epidemic of obesity. Americans are eating more and exercising less. Our waistbands are expanding as are our medical bills, as the extra weight adds to the number of new patients diagnosed with diabetes, high blood pressure, varicose veins, and other preventable diseases and conditions. Simply put, Americans are eating themselves sick.

concluding sentence

So each support paragraph will have a topic sentence to begin with, support details and examples, and a concluding sentence.

Exercise 12-4: Continue with the topic you chose in Exercise 12-3. Draft two support paragraphs for this topic.

First support paragraph:

Second support paragraph:

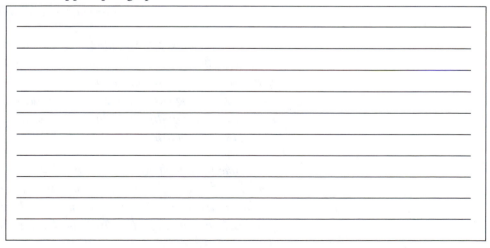

WRITING THE CONCLUDING PARAGRAPH

The concluding paragraph summarizes the points from the body paragraphs. The paragraph often begins with a sentence that restates or is tied to the thesis statement. Then some general sentences that review your points of view follow to sum up your point. Try to leave the reader thinking about the topic. An effective conclusion ties all your points together and convinces the reader that you have made your point. Note: No new information or data should be added to the conclusion paragraph, as the point is to end the essay.

Americans have found themselves living the American dream—fast car, busy life, and quick food. Our problem is not the lack of food but the nutrient value of the food that we ingest. The high-fat diet coupled with the lack of adequate exercise has positioned the public for a health crisis—obesity costs more in healthcare issues. Most importantly, this disease is preventable. Shouldn't we be more conscious of what we are eating and what we choose to do with our health?

EXERCISE 12-5: Write a concluding paragraph that continues your essay from 12-3 and 12-4.

____
____
____
____
____
____
____
____
____
____

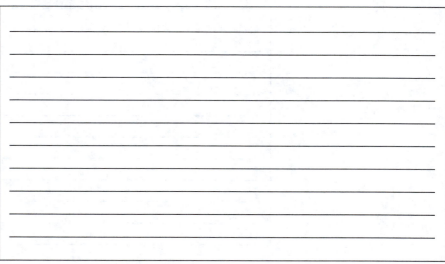

For the Health's Sake

Food, cooking, and shopping opportunities meet us around every street corner and shopping aisle. We are a society of consumers, food-wise and money-wise. Television shows and glossy magazine covers encourage cooking and eating. Overeating has become an epidemic because Americans have lost their desire to consume healthy foods in limited portions, and the majority of Americans have a weight problem.

Americans no longer limit their intake to nutritional needs; instead, Americans buy or order more food than they can or should eat. Portions have been doubled or tripled by biggy fries and supersized meals. In addition to this, we eat fiberless, fatty foods that offer diminished food value. Often the meats are eaten on the run, in our cars, or at our desks, so there is no sense of consumption durations or quantities. Thus, Americans consume excessive amounts of food, yet still find themselves hungering for another bite.

Overeating in America has created an epidemic of obesity. Americans are eating more and exercising less. Our waistbands are expanding as are our medical bills, as the extra weight adds to the number of new patients diagnosed with diabetes, high blood pressure, varicose veins, and other preventable diseases and conditions. Simply put, Americans are eating themselves sick.

Americans have found themselves living the American dream—fast car, busy life, and quick food. Our problem is not the lack of food but the nutrient value of the food that we ingest. The high-fat diet coupled with the lack of adequate exercise has positioned the public for a health crisis—obesity costs more in healthcare issues. Most importantly, this disease is preventable. Shouldn't we be more conscious of what we are eating and what we choose to do with our health?

EXAMPLE OF ANOTHER COMPLETED ESSAY

How Do You Define Success?

People measure success differently. Some people mark their successes by the things that they buy and own. Others think that success is having a happy family. Success for me is measured by my work because I love to help people, and I believe that I can make a difference in their lives.

I love to help people, so when I work with others, I feel great. To feel that I have been helpful to another person allows me to feel successful. One example is when I help a student learn how to do a math problem. The success I feel is a result of the success the other person is having. So helping people is a large part of my own feelings about success.

My success means I can make a difference in students' lives. So many times, students feel that writing and math are too difficult to learn or too hard to improve because they have learned these skills before. If I provide students with step-by-step instructions and allow them time to practice, they will learn. Once the learning begins, there is nothing to stop them from being successful. Thus, their learning makes a difference in their lives and contributes to my feeling successful.

So success for me is defined by my ability to help other people improve their lives by learning. When others have a feeling of success, I also feel their success and my own success. Deciding on my own personal definition of success took me many years of hard work and soul searching to find happiness within myself. For me, success is not about lots of money, new clothes, or a shiny car. Instead, success is about working to help others feel success.

Name ______________________________

Self-Checklist for Essay Writing

After completing the essay, check each of the tasks completed:

Introductory Paragraph

______ I have several general sentences related to the topic beginning the paragraph.

______ I have placed the thesis statement last in the paragraph.

______ I have written the main-idea sentence so that it includes *because* or *by* to introduce the two reasons supporting my opinion.

______ I am sure that the main-idea sentence addresses or answers the essay topic or question.

Support Paragraphs

______ I used the reasons from the thesis statement to form the topic sentences of the support paragraphs.

______ I have given specific reasons, details, and examples to support each support paragraph's topic sentence.

______ I have provided a concluding sentence for each support paragraph.

Conclusion

_____ I have written a summary sentence that restates my main point.

_____ I have provided a review or a thought about the topic for the reader to consider about the topic.

_____ I have left the reader with the sense that my essay is complete.

_____ I have not added any new information in this paragraph.

Final Proofreading and Revision

_____ I have read the entire essay.

_____ I have check for spelling errors and corrected them.

_____ I have checked for correct punctuation.

_____ I have answered the essay question.

Peer Edit

_____ I have asked ______________________ to read and edit my essay.

EXERCISE 12-6: Choose *one* of the following topics and draft an essay.

1. Why are more and more nurses being charged in criminal court for their mishandling of patient care?
2. What is the most important advice for any new parent to know about caring for an infant?
3. Explain what impact diet has on mental, physical, and emotional health.
4. Discuss one of the social stigmas attached to illnesses such as AIDS, tuberculosis, or alcoholism.
5. Explain how ethnicity plays a role in attaining health services.
6. What is a pet peeve that you have about doctor's offices?
7. Is our insurance system helping or hindering healthcare services for elderly?
8. What two improvements would you like to see in your healthcare plan?
9. Why are people into quick fixes for their healthcare issues?
10. How can the general public be motivated to exercise more and eat better?

USING ESSAY WRITING SKILLS FOR COURSE PAPERS

The same principles for writings essays can generally be applied to writing research papers or other academic papers. It is important to follow copyright laws, avoid plagiarism, and to always give credit whenever materials have been borrowed from another source.

ANNOTATED BIBLIOGRAPHIES

An annotated bibliography includes the works cited in the text along with a brief evaluative description of the material. The evaluative comments may or may not be in complete sentences. An annotated bibliography can be arranged alphabetically by author, by subject, or by chronological order.

Students sometimes ask what should be included in an annotated bibliography. Some ideas include:

1. description of the content
2. the usefulness of the material found within the text
3. the background of the author
4. limitations of the materials presented by the text
5. the organization of the content
6. the reader's reaction to the content or text

Here are some examples:

Ping, W. (2002). *Aching for beauty: Footbinding in China.* New York: Anchor Books. Ping details the cultural and political details behind footbinding in China. This account is a provocative and thought-provoking comprehensive look at the custom.

Willet, W. (2003). *Eat, drink, and be healthy.* New York: Free Press. The author presents the information in an easy-to-read format supported by data and facts supported by research. The text is very readable as Willets connects diet and health.

Exercise 12-7: Using a professional journal, locate one article of interest. After reading the article, write an annotated bibliography.

____

____

____

____

____

____

Go to the library and locate a book in your field. Then draft an annotated bibliography of a chapter or portion of the text.

____

____

____

____

____

____

Use one of your textbooks for a course and draft an annotated bibliography.

____

____

____

____

____

____

Sometimes annotated bibliographies are longer and more detailed. An example from a nursing student is provided below:

Bianchi-Sand, S. (2003, December). It takes a team to prevent errors. *American Journal of Nursing, 103*(12), 1–4. Retrieved May 21, 2004, from http://www.nursingworld.org/AJN/2003/dec/issues.htm

This article states how to deal with preventable medical errors. The article is well written and organized.

In "It Takes a Team to Prevent Errors" in *American Journal of Nursing*, Susan Bianchi-Sand reports that better communication among healthcare professionals is a key component to avoid human mistakes when providing patient care. In order to provide safe patient care, the nurses and doctors need to have clear and correct communication. Healthcare is not the only industry that is prone to human mistakes. Hence, the article states a strategy that the airline industry is using to avoid tragedies associated with preventable human mistakes.

According to this article, medical errors cause about 98,000 deaths in America each year. The main cause for this tragedy is poor communication between nurses and doctors. Unless all doctors value the nurses' inputs, knowledge, and judgment on patient care, more lives are at stake. Doctors need to be team players. Nurses should be encouraged to actively participate in the patient care by speaking up about what they think is the best care for their client.

The author points out how health professionals ought to learn from the airline industry. The airline industry has developed a program called crew resource management (CRM) training. The training is designed to equip crew members on how to work together as a team by using different talents of each person. In this program, the captain works with flight attendants to ensure the safety of the passengers. In conclusion, since the core element of a healthcare system is the patient, the nurses and doctors should work as a team to prevent errors. This article is relevant to nursing because it shows that nurses' input is significant to safeguard patients, and nurses need to be encouraged to be an advocate for their patients.

Written by Azeb Zeleke, LPN student

RESEARCH PAPERS

Research papers are essays that respond to a question or an assignment that requires research of some sort. Most research papers require a set number of citations or works consulted.

REFERENCE CITATIONS

These types of papers have in-text reference citations that provide information on the source of the information. Students are asked to choose either the MLA (Modern Language Association) style guide or the APA (American Pscyhological Association) style guide and then follow that format for the paper. Sometimes instructors add their own requirements to one of these style guides. In any case, select either of the style guides and follow its rules for documentation.

Any library will provide the style guides. Online references are plenty and very helpful.

Any Internet search will provide a wide variety of reference sources. Two resources are www.mla.org and www.apastyle.org.

Additional information on these style guides can be found at:

- www.healthlinks.washington.edu/hsl/styleguides.apa.html
- www.crk.umn.edu/library/links/apa5th.htm
- www.libs.uga.edu/ref/mlastyle.html
- http://owl.english.purdue.edu/handouts/research/r_mla.html
- http://www.columbia.edu/cu/cup/cgos/idx_basic.html

These sources will help provide the information that will help format the paper.

A word about plagiarism: Do not do it. Plagiarism is using any material from another source without proper citation. Sometimes students question what to cite. In general, follow these guidelines: Cite if the information is

1. another person's research, data, idea, or opinion
2. another's person speech or written work
3. any facts, data, or details that are not common or general knowledge

Common knowledge is information that is known by a lot of people and written in a wide variety of places. For example, the United States is made up of 50 states. We know this as a society; thus, there is no need to cite it.

Decide how to cite the work based on what you are using in the text. Overciting is better than not citing information from others.

Type of Information Used	Use This Type of Citation
Direct quotation	Use quotation marks around the quote and an in-text reference and a complete citation on the reference page.
Longer piece from which you borrow information, but paraphrase the information	Use an in-text reference and a complete citation on the reference page.
Graphics, data, statistics	Use an in-text reference and a complete citation on the reference page.

Use both the in-text references and references at the end of the paper to ensure that any material that is not solely yours is given a citation entry. The chart below details the most common formats to use. Other more specific information on citations can be gained by referring to the above websites or a hard copy of the style guides.

Reference Sheet for APA Citation Formatting

Entry Type	In-text Citation	References (separate page at end of the paper)
Book, 1–2 authors	(Sorokie, 2004)	Sorokie, A. M. (2004). *Gut wisdom: Understanding and improving your digestive health.* Franklin Lakes, NJ: New Page Books.

Book, 3+ authors	(Easton et al., 1991)	Easton, P. S., Harter, C., Higgins, C., & Mengel, M. (1991). *Nutrition care of people with diabetes mellitus.* New York: Food Products Press.
Book chapter	(South, 1996)	South, V. (1996). *Migraine: Everything you need to know* (pp 1–16). Toronto: Key Porter Books.
Book, editor	(Gersh, 2000)	Gersh, B. J. (Eds). (2000). *Mayo Clinic heart book.* New York: William Morrow.
Journal, 1 author, paginated	(Singla, 2004)	Singla, D. (2004, April). Nonprescription treatment of allergic rhinitis. *Pharmacy Times*, 40–41.
Journal, 2+ authors, paginated	(Boothby, Doering, & Jaco, 2004)	Boothby, L., Doering, P., & Jaco, V. (2004, July/August). When prescription drugs go over the counter: Where are the boundaries? *Journal of Pharmacy Technology, 20*, 215–220.
Journal, electronic	(Leishmaniasis, 2005)	Leishmaniasis vaccine: Drug sensitive leishmania vaccine developed. (2005, March 29). *Science Letter.* Retrieved March 30, 2005 from Proquest Database.
Internet, from print	(Bianchi-Sands, 2003)	Bianchi-Sands, S. (2003). It takes a team to prevent errors [Electronic version]. *American Journal of Nursing, 103*, 1–4.
Magazine	(Zouali, 2005)	Zouali, M. (2005, March). Taming lupus. *Scientific American, 292*, 71–77.
Newspaper	(Powelson, 2004)	Powelson, R. (2004, December 30). Go slow with weight loss, nutrition experts advise. *The Seattle Post-Intelligencer,* p. A2.

Based on the *Publication Manual of the American Psychological Association*, 5th edition, 2001.

EXERCISE 12-8: Use the following information to make an APA-formatted reference citation.

1. Frederick Fell Publishers, Inc. By Marianne Pilgrim Calabrese. Hollywood, California. 2004. So you want to be a Nurse? pp 23–26

____

____

____

2. JADA–Journal of the American Dental Association. November 2004. pp. 1537–1542. The integration of clinical research into dental therapies: The role of the astute clinician. Volume 135. Sharon M. Gordon, DDS, MPH, PhD. Raymond A. Dionne, DDS, PhD.

____

____

____

3. Asthma Treatment Guidelines and Medications pp 32–37, April. Pharmacy Times. April. Lauren S. Schlesselman. (2000, April).

___

___

___

4. Janice M. Boutotte, RN, CS, MS. Volume 29, Number 3, 1999, March. pp 34–39. Nursing 99. Keeping TB in check.

___

___

___

5. 2000. Salvatore Tocci, New York. Franklin Watts. Down Syndrome.

___

___

___

Reference Sheet for MLA Citation Formatting

Entry Type	In-Text Citation	References (separate page at end of the paper)
Book, 1 author	(Sorokie 34)	Sorokie, Alyce M. Gut Wisdom: Understanding and Improving Your Digestive Health. Franklin Lakes, NJ: New Page Books, 2004.
Book, 4+ authors	(Easton et al. 27)	Easton, Penelope S., et al. Nutrition Care of People with Diabetes Mellitus: A Nutritional Reference for Health Professionals. New York: Haworth Press Inc., 1991.
Book chapter	(South 13)	South,Valerie. Migraine: Everything You Need to Know. Toronto: Key Porter Books, 1996.
Book, editor	(Gersh 104)	Gersh, Bernard J., ed. Mayo Clinic Heart Book. New York: William Morrow, 2000.
Journal, 1 author, paginated	(Singla 41)	Singla, Dana L. "Nonprescription Treatment of Allergic Rhinitis." Pharmacy Times, April 2004: 40–41.
Journal, 2+ authors, paginated	(Boothby et al. 215)	Boothby, Lisa A., Paul L. Doering, & Vi T. Jaco. "When Prescription Drugs Go Over the Counter: Where are the Boundaries?" Journal of Pharmacy Technology, 20 (2004): 215–220.
Journal, electronic	(Leishmaniasis par. 2) [See section 6.4.1 of the *MLA Handbook* for more information.]	"Leishmaniasis Vaccine: Drug Sensitive Leishmania Vaccine Developed." 29 Mar. 2005. Online posting. Science Letter. 5 Apr. 2005 Proquest Database.

Internet, from print	(Bianchi-Sands, par. 3) [See section 6.4.1of the *MLA Hand book* for more information.]	Bianchi-Sands, Susan. "It Takes a Team to Prevent Errors." American Journal of Nursing, Dec. 2003. 3 Sept. 2005 <http:www.nursingworld.org/AJN/2003/dec/issues.htm>.
Magazine	(Zouali 71)	Zouali, Moncef. "Taming Lupus." Scientific American, 292, March 2005: 71–77.
Newspaper	(Powelson A2)	Powelson, Richard. "Go Slow with Weight Loss, Nutrition Experts Advise." The Seattle Post-Intelligencer 30 Dec. 2004: A2.
Web page	(University of Washington, par. 4) [See section 6.4.1 of the *MLA Hand book* for more information.]	University of Washington. "Healthlinks: APA Style Guide." 2 Mar. 1999. Online posting. 28 Mar. 2005 <http://healthlinks.washinton.edu/hsl/styleguides apa.htm>.

Based on the *MLA Handbook for Writers of Research Papers* (6th edition).

EXERCISE 12-9: Use the following information to make an MLA-formatted reference citation.

1. Frederick Fell Publishers, Inc. By Marianne Pilgrim Calabrese. Hollywood, California. 2004. So you want to be a Nurse? pp 23–26.

 ____

 ____

 ____

2. JADA–Journal of the American Dental Association. November 2004. pp. 1537–1542. The integration of clinical research into dental therapies: The role of the astute clinician. Volume 135. Sharon M. Gordon, DDS, MPH, PhD. Raymond A. Dionne, DDS, PhD.

 ____

 ____

 ____

3. Asthma Treatment: Guidelines and Medications. pp 32–37. April. Pharmacy Times. April. Lauren S. Schlesselman. April 2004.

 ____

 ____

 ____

4. Janice M. Boutotte, RN, CS, MS. Volume 29 Number 3, 1999 March. pp 34–39. Nursing 99. Keeping TB in check.

 ____

 ____

 ____

5. 2000. Salvatore Tocci, New York. Franklin Watts. Down Syndrome.

____

____

____

Research papers vary in length and style. Each has a thesis and supporting evidence. Below are two samples. Notice the difference in styles and levels of formality.

As family sizes begin to decrease in America, pets, dogs in particular, have sometimes become like surrogate children. American strive to be the best pet owners possible, waking up early to exercise their dogs and making sure that their puppies are vaccinated and examined on time. As a former veterinary technician, I have witnessed firsthand the love that compels owners to spend hundreds of dollars at veterinary clinics, hoping to give their pets health that will increase their longevity.

Between their baths, vaccinations, and behavioral medications, American pets' needs are beginning to rival American children's needs. Sadly, more and more pets are becoming victims of diseases that cannot be cured with a simple vaccination and that mirror the human diseases that plague Americans today. Such diseases, which include cancer, epilepsy, hip dysplasia, thyroid disease, allergies, and heart disease, mainly affect purebred dogs; these conditions are usually caused by inbreeding, which leads us to believe that genetics is a key to preventing these diseases. Genetic studies, underway around the nation, may discover the way to alleviate our pets' suffering and perhaps to help humans along the way. But one wonders if genetics is the main culprit. What about the animal's upbringing and home environment?

Most researchers and veterinarians assume that hip dysplasia is caused fifty percent by genetics and fifty percent by environment. I recently read an article that refuted this assumption and awakened me to what a truly good owner would do for her pet. The article, by M. C. Wakeman, D.V.M., reveals the results of some clinical findings that show that hip dyplasia is largely related to the growth rate and the amount of exercise in dogs. Thus, "there is no such thing as *congenital* unilateral hip dysplasia, but only *acquired* unilateral hip dysplasia" (Wakeman, 2001). In the study, the researchers maximized the exercise of one group of large-breed puppies while confining exercise to only an hour or two a day for the second group. Both groups were offered equal amounts of food. The first group grew slowly because their energy from their food went into their exercise, whereas the second group grew quickly because their food energy was unnecessary for exercise, so it made them grow. The researchers concluded that the second group's dogs grew "much too quickly for their biology to keep up" (Wakeman, 2001). Furthermore, these dogs' rear limbs grew more quickly than their front limbs, which reduced the mechanical leverage that the muscles exerted and made the puppies more susceptible to injury. In addition, their muscle tone was "a small fraction of that of a puppy which plays with other active dogs all day long" (Wakeman, 2001).

Although these are the findings of only one study, the implications of the article moved me. Humans sometimes unfairly expect animals to live like humans. Dogs, like humans, function best when they live a physically and mentally stimulating life. Thus, a dog that is cooped up all day long with unlimited access to food and with little mental action will likely not only become a victim of a multitude of health problems but also lose its mental vigor. Thus, their health conditions are not caused exclusively by genetics. The genetics comes first; however, once the dog is born, its quality of life is determined by its environment within its genetic limitations.

Thus two critical factors, genetics and environment, determine the quality of our animal's lives. If we truly do care about our pets as much as we say, then it is our responsibility to buy or adopt animals that are not inbred and to choose to provide an environment for our pets that fits their needs as animals. I realize that if everyone followed these two guidelines, far fewer people would own pets. But maybe that's the most responsible decision to make if we truly loved our pets.

Wakeman, M.C. (2001, July 16). Unilateral hip dysplasia. Retrieved Oct. 10, 2001, from www.showdogssupersite.com/hips.html.

Written by Jade Benjamin-Chung, UC Berkeley Public Health Student

The following essay is a research paper written for a nursing course. The student was asked to research a current topic and write a paper in APA format. The paper discusses the issues surrounding organ donation in the United States.

Jackie Elms

Medical/Surgical Nursing

Monday, February 12, 2004

Organ Donation: The Incentive Debate

According to Dykstra, there are nearly 70,000 people on a waiting list for various organs in the United States. Approximately 150 people are added each day, and approximately 50 people die each day having never received their needed organ. There are many ethical, cultural, and legal challenges to organ donation. As a nurse, you must be sensitive to these challenges and promote organ donation appropriately via patient and family teaching and/or advocate for patients and their families when the question arises whether or not to donate their organs. Worldwide attention is being focused on this organ shortage, and many healthcare professionals, policymakers, and ethicists have been brainstorming ideas to increase the rate of donations. This paper will discuss some of these ideas and their challenges.

Currently in the United States we follow the "opt-in" approach to organ donation via a national program through the Department of Motor Vehicles.

People can indicate their desire to donate their organs when they renew their driver's license. By placing a sticker on his or her driver's license that says "organ donor," a person has opted-in and agrees to donate organs. However, in the event of an accident, if the patient's family is not aware of his or her wishes, the family can decline to donate. As a nurse, it is important for you to encourage the healthy patients you see every day to discuss their wishes with their family members now. Our culture in America is hesitant to discuss death. We feel as though "it can't happen to us" or "I don't have to worry about that now," but accidents happen, and it is important to make your wishes known. Educate your patients that any adult, age 18 and over, can create a legal document called a Living Will.

This document gives family and healthcare personnel specific instructions to resuscitate (full code) or not to resuscitate (DNAR) in the event of cardiac or respiratory distress. In addition, in the event of a patient's death, it gives voice to his or her wishes for the body, its organs, and its resting-place.

Spain, which has the highest rate of donation in the world, takes the opposite approach. They follow an "opt-out" program. You *are* an organ donor unless you specify otherwise. The family of the deceased is neither consulted nor can legally object to the donations. As a nurse in Spain, the challenge would not be to encourage donation but to support the family members after the fact.

A hot debate is brewing out of Canada, according to Kondro, whether online recruitment for organ donation is ethical. Altruistic live donations have been discouraged in the past due to the health risk for the donors and the risk that donors are selling pieces of themselves, which is against a federal law on organ trafficking. However, ever-increasing numbers of patients waiting for donations have pressured some of their transplant centers to accept live donor organs. Online sources like the nonprofit site Livingdonorsonline.org have successfully connected patients to altruistic donors who are willing to "give" life. Another site, Matchingdonors.com, charges patients $295 per month to post profiles and pleas for organs.

These types of sites prompted the United Network for Organ Sharing, the agency that manages the American organ supply, to argue that the principles of organ donation and the fair distribution of these organs are being undermined. That is to say, the way the organs are distributed now is according to who is the sickest, not by who wants to give to whom and who can pay more or get away with profiting from organ trafficking.

Another set of models under the investigation suggests that the U.S. government become involved and create a financial incentive program to increase donation rates. In this model, the government would institute either an income tax credit or funeral expense reimbursement for promised donation. The problem with this and other incentives is that not all organs are good organs. A person with HIV or hepatitis C cannot donate organs and therefore would not qualify for this program; how would the government legally investigate that without invading the privacy of the donor?

According to Salladay, a decreased donor can be categorized into one of two groups, either a brain-dead individual or a nonheartbeating donor, both of whose organs are then harvested and distributed to waiting patients. It is unethical for the medical community to facilitate death in order to harvest an organ. It is also currently unethical to knowingly allow a donor to sell parts of him- or herself for money. As a nurse, you may be asked to assist in a "harvest procedure." Salladay wants you to be aware of your hospital's policies and procedures for organ harvesting and donation. If you have any concerns as to whether the procedure is ethical or within policy limits, speak to your nurse-manager immediately.

Organ donation is an important issue on which you, as a nurse, can be very instrumental in affecting change. The public is uneducated about the benefits and the risks. Many lives would be saved if more people would elect to be organ donors.

References

Dykstra, A. (2004). Should incentives be used to increase organ donation? *Plastic Surgical Nursing, 24*(2), 70–74.

Kondro, W. (2005). Debate of online recruitment of organ donors. *Canadian Medical Association Journal, 172*(2), 165–166.

Salladay, S. A. (2004). Organ donation: Defining death. *Nursing 2004, 34*(8), 10.

UNIT PROOFREADING EXERCISES

Read the following annotated bibliography and make changes in punctuation, spelling, and format. Cross the errors out neatly and replace with the corrections.

S. Trossman. (February 2004,). Want a safer patient care. *American journal of Nursing*, 104(2)
In this article the author states improving working conditions of nurses produce quality patient care. This is organized and well written article.

In the February 2004 issue of *American Journal of Nursing* an article entitled, "Want Safe Patient Care"? Susan Trossman notes that the (IOM) Institute of Medicine puts emphasize on the improving working conditions of nurses to provide a better patient care. Both IOM and (AN) American Nursing Association acknowledge that proper patient care is in danger when there is understaffing makes it difficult for the nurse to provide quality bed side care when working long hours. Therefore the

IOM points out recommendations that could solve these problems.

The IOM advices that hospitals and long term facilities inforce a staffing level for every shift and unit that meet the needs of each patient such as scheduled procedure, emergency care, or discharging practices. Cross-trained staff members can be valuable assets for this flexibility. The nursing staff should play an active role in designing and implementing a staffing system that will ensure patient safety. The IOM also addresses overtime by recommending state governments to ban 12-hour shifts. In addition IMO encourages nursing schools and health organization to teach the danger of fatigue caused by prolonged working hours on patient safety.

The article has value to nursing because it shows the great danger of inadequate patient care caused by unsatisfactory working conditions of nurses. Plus, the nurse must be an advocate for the patient whenever the patient's needs are not meet because of understaffing. In conclusion this articles is importance because it deals with the solutions to solve poor working conditions of nurse to provide quality patient care.

Adapted from Azeb Zeleke, LPN Student

UNIT REVISION EXERCISES

Revise the following annotated bibliography. Neatly rearrange the information or make the corrections.

Trossman, S. (2004, February). *American journal of Nursing,* Want a safer patient care. 104(2).

In this article the author states improving working conditions of nurses produce quality patient care. The article is organized and well written.

In the February 2004 monthly issue of *American Journal of Nursing* an article that is entitled, "Want Safe Patient Care?" Susan notes that the Institute of Medicine (IOM) puts emphasize on the improving working conditions of nurses to provide a best patient care. Both IOM and American Nursing Association (ANA) acknowledge that proper patient care is in danger when there is understaffing made it difficult for the nurse to provide quality bed side care when working long hours. Therefore, the IOM points out suggestions and recommendations that could solve these problems.

The IOM advises that hospitals and long term facilities enforce a staffing level for every shifts and units that meet the needs of each patient such as scheduled procedure, emergency care, or discharging practices. Cross-trained staff members can be valuable assets for this flexibility. The nursing staff should play an active role in designing and implementing a staffing system that will ensure patient safety. The IOM also addresses overtime by recommending state governments to ban 12 hours shifts. In addition, IOM encourages nursing schools and health organization to teach the danger of fatigue caused by prolonged working hours on patient safety.

The article has to nursing value because it shows the great danger of inadequate patient care caused by unsatisfactory working conditions of nurses. Plus, the nurse must be an advocate for the patients wherever the patient's needs are not meet because of understaffing. In conclusion, this article is important because of the fact that it deals with the solutions to solve poor working conditions of nurse to provide quality patient care.

Adapted from Azeb Zeleke, LPN Student

UNIT EXTENSIONS

1. Develop a healthcare survey for the class or the student body. Distribute the survey and then collect and tabulate the data. Draft a report of your findings using the information that you collected. Develop graphics and general trends of the group that were surveyed.
2. Draft ten writing prompts for research papers that might be of interest to student in your field.
3. Go to www.apastyle.org and study the format instructions for reference citations in this style guide. Then locate ten different reference citations that follow the instructions for APA formatting. You might use medical journals, textbooks, and the Internet as the source. Type these collected ten citations on a handout to use as a crib sheet for future reference.

UNIT 12 SELF-CHECK

Write a three-page research paper on a current healthcare issue, a specific drug, a medical organization, or a public policy. Use APA formatting and type the paper. Provide at least five reference citations. Ask a peer to edit it for you. Make revisions. Submit it to the instructor for scoring. Use the following Self-Check list for research papers in your proofreading and revision.

Research Writing Checklist

After completing the essay, check each of the tasks completed:

Introductory Paragraph

______ I have several general sentences related to the topic beginning the paragraph.

______ I have placed the thesis statement last in the paragraph.

______ I have written the thesis statement so that the reader is clear on the research question I am answering and the content of the paper.

______ I am sure that the main-idea sentence addresses or answers the essay topic or question.

Support Paragraphs

______ I used the reasons from the thesis statement to form the topic sentences of the support paragraphs.

______ I have given specific reasons, details, and examples to support each support paragraph's topic sentence.

______ I have provided a concluding sentence for each support paragraph.

Conclusion

______ I have written a summary sentence that restates my main point.

______ I have provided a review or a thought about the topic for the reader to consider.

______ I have left the reader with the sense that my essay is complete.

______ I have not added any new information in this paragraph.

Citations

______ I have given credit in citations for all borrowed information.

______ I have included in-text citations.

______ I have introduced all quotations.

______ I have used correct punctuation with my in-text citations.

______ I have created a reference citation at the end of the paper for each source used.

Final Proofreading and Revision

______ I have read the entire essay.

______ I have checked for spelling errors and corrected them.

______ I have checked for correct punctuation.

______ I have answered the essay question.

Peer Edit

______ I have asked ________________________________ to read and edit my essay.

Answer Key

UNIT 1: GRAMMAR BASICS

EXERCISE 1-1 Fill in the chart with the correct form to make these words singular or plural

Singular	Plural
carcinoma	carcinomata; carcinomas
ganglion	ganglia
apex	apices
diagnosis	diagnoses
pleura	pleurae

EXERCISE 1-2 Read the passage below; then underline each noun.

Many herbs and vitamins have shown new hope for treating diabetes. There is some concern for the safety and efficacy of herbal remedies. It may be too soon for experts to make recommendations about most of these herbs and vitamins, but the medical community is showing some interest in these alternative approaches to healthcare.

EXERCISE 1-3 Write sentences with the following common nouns. These are sample sentences only. Yours will vary.

1. pediatrics

   Pediatrics is the specialty of treating childhood diseases and conditions.

2. acne

   Many teens experience acne.

3. tension

   The tension in the room was unbearable.

4. surgeon

   The surgeon was scrubbing for surgery.

5. cancer

   Cancer treatment options are increasing with research.

Exercise 1-4 Underline the subject in the following sentences. These are sample sentences only. Yours will vary.

1. The amputation—a partial or complete removal of a limb—was performed by the medical team in the military hospital.
2. A fracture indicates a breakage of a bone by disease or trauma.
3. His condition of gout has caused acute arthritis and joint inflammation.
4. Your insulin, used to treat diabetes, will lower your glucose levels.
5. Her osteoplasty is scheduled for early June.

Exercise 1-5 Complete the chart with specialists and fields.

Specialist	Field/Practice of Specialty	Type of Care Provided
endocrinologist	endocrinology	treatment of disease of the endocrine gland
anesthesiologist	anesthesiology	administration of anesthesia to patients to create partial or complete loss of sensation
pharmacist	pharmacology	dispensing of prescribed medications
immunologist	immunology	treatment of diseases of the immune system
endodontist	endodontics	diagnosis, treatment, and prevention of diseases of the dental pulp and surrounding tissues
otolaryngologist	otolaryngology	treatment of ear, nose, and throat diseases
orthodontist	orthodontics	prevention and correction of misaligned teeth
ophthalmologist	ophthalmology	treatment of the disorders of the eye
gynecologist	gynecology	treatment of the diseases specific to women
osteopath	osteopathy	treatment of diseases of the bone

Exercise 1-6 Use these pronouns in sentences. These are sample sentences only. Yours will vary.

1. our

   Our family doctor is Dr. Marian Ohashi.

2. whose

   The nurse asked whose form this was.

3. they

   They are counseling the family about the patient's options.

4. yours

   John's treatment plan is ready; yours will be prepared later today.

5. her

   Her preference is for day surgery.

EXERCISE 1-7 Write sentences with these pronouns.

1. everything

   Everything is ready in the resident's room.

2. each

   Each of the family members saw her before surgery.

3. few

   Few want to become ill.

4. most

   Most of the research has occurred within the past ten years.

5. half

   Half of the medical students are now women.

EXERCISE 1-8 Identify the verb and underline the verb type for each sentence. Then underline the correct modifying word in parentheses for each sentence.

Verb Type	
1. Action or Linking Verb	The disturbed resident yelled (loud, loudly).
2. Action or Linking Verb	The LPN student performed (good, well) at his clinical site.
3. Action or Linking Verb	The doctor could (sure, surely) order the tests.
4. Action or Linking Verb	The surgical team looked (tired, tiredly) after the 12 hours of work.
5. Action or Linking Verb	The family seems (unhappy, unhappily) with the diagnosis.
6. Action or Linking Verb	Today, the patient felt (good, well) after the examination and medical tests.

EXERCISE 1-9 Write sentences that incorporate these verbs. Refer to unit glossary for definitions of these words. These are sample sentences only. Yours will vary.

1. excise

   The surgeon excised the tumor.

2. cauterize

   The dentist cauterizes the sores to promote healing.

3. diagnose

   The radiologist diagnosed her cancer.

4. incise

   The doctor will incise the vein and make the repair.

5. instruct

   The registered nurse instructs the assistant in patient care.

EXERCISE 1-10 Read the passage below, then underline each adjective.

Recently, the medical community has discussed the need for all people to reduce the fat in their diets. The fast food industry has supersized portions that encourage people to overeat. Today many people are reducing the amount of food that they ingest. By reducing their intake, individuals hope to extend their healthy years.

EXERCISE 1-11 Write a sentence with each adjective. Refer to unit glossary for definitions of these words. These are sample sentences only. Yours will vary.

1. cardiac

   The cardiac arrest lasted almost 55 seconds.

2. dermal

   The dermal abrasion needs cleansing.

3. salivary

   Salivary glands produce saliva, which helps human beings digest food.

4. muscular

   His muscular build indicates that he has done strength-building exercises.

5. gastric

   Gastric bypass surgery is a serious procedure to consider.

EXERCISE 1-12 Read the passage below; then underline each adverb.

Phoenix, Arizona, has a very big problem this year. According to health officials, the state is the only state where the mosquito-borne West Nile virus has already reached an epidemic. Arizona has a lot of standing water in the form of pools and irrigation ditches. This water effectively harbors these insects. So far, there have been 290 cases of West Nile virus in Arizona this year. State officials are very worried that as many as 300,000 Arizonians might have the virus; they may not know it yet. The officials are carefully monitoring the situation.

EXERCISE 1-13 Use the following adverbs in a sentence. These are sample sentences only. Yours will vary.

1. rather

   The patient was rather upset by the procedure.

2. here

   Here are the files that you requested, Dr. Brim.

3. not

   The decision is not mine to make.

4. then

   The patient then asked for the chaplain.

5. cautiously

   The girl cautiously held her new baby brother.

EXERCISE 1-14 Read the passage below; then underline each prepositional phrase.

A certified nursing assistant (CNA) is an entry-level caregiver. The job duties <u>of a CNA</u> are varied. Much <u>of the difficult tasks</u> are completed <u>by these dedicated and caring individuals</u>. They are <u>trained in personal hygiene</u>, first aid, care giving, bed making, and feeding techniques. <u>From morning to night</u>, patients rely <u>on their assistance</u>. Sometimes, a senior citizen may have only a CNA who pays attention <u>to his or her daily needs.</u> Thus, the value <u>of the role</u> <u>of the certified nursing assistant</u> should not be taken <u>for granted.</u>

EXERCISE 1-15 Write sentences that include these prepositional phrases. These are sample sentences only. Yours will vary.

1. beside the examination table

   Beside the examination table were magazines and educational materials.

2. for the laboratory procedure

   For the laboratory procedure, a new technician requested assistance.

3. in trauma cases

   In trauma cases, families need to become educated about recovery.

4. under the doctor's care

   Grandfather is under the doctor's care for hypertension.

5. among the bandages

   Among the bandages was the sign of blood seepage.

EXERCISE 1-16 Read each sentence. Underline the conjunction and write the type of conjunction on the blank line. Use these labels: coordinating conjunction (cc), correlative conjunction (corr), or subordinating conjunction (sc).

1. <u>Because</u> depression is prominent on college campuses, college counselors are using more interventions to assist students. <u>sc</u>
2. The students wanted to research the disease, <u>so</u> the professor gained access to the data for them. <u>cc</u>
3. <u>The more</u> she worked on her medical terminology, <u>the more</u> proficient she became as a medical receptionist. <u>corr</u>
4. Lyme disease can make some people feel fatigued and in pain, <u>while</u> others suffer depression, anxiety, and memory loss. <u>sc</u>
5. The disease started with a rash, <u>and</u> it is followed with flulike symptoms. <u>cc</u>

EXERCISE 1-17 Use each of the conjunctions in a sentence. These are sample sentences only. Yours will vary.

1. while

   While the family went home to rest, their friends stayed in the hospital room.

2. as if

   She looked as if she would cry at any moment.

3. but

   He was tired, but he felt relieved at the latest news about his wife's condition.

4. before

   Before we see the doctor, we need to go to the blood work laboratory.

5. not only . . . but also

   Not only is she frustrated by her weight, but she is also discouraged by her health condition.

EXERCISE 1-18 Add an ending or suffix to each word to make the desired form of the word. Endings to be used are *–ment, –ed, –ate, –ion,* and *–tic,* to complete the table. Fill in the correct form of the word. If none exists, use an *X* in the box to indicate that none exists. Some words may change spelling.

Noun	Verb	Adjective
depression	depress	depressed
vaccination	vaccinate	vaccinated
medication; medicine	medicate	medicated
incision	incise	incised
enrichment	enrich	enriched
spasm	X	spastic

EXERCISE 1-19 Complete the following prepositional phrases.

1. of the skin
2. against the wall
3. except for the relatives
4. after the surgery
5. between the teeth

EXERCISE 1-20 Underline each verb and verb phrase.

The hospital assistant is making Mr. Anderson's bed and preparing (is preparing) for his return. The patient is completing some X-rays on the first floor. Then he will return for a brief rest. Thereafter, he will complete a session of occupational therapy on the fifth floor. Rehabilitation requires daily exercise and adherence to a specific plan. Mr. Anderson is usually motivated to complete his exercises each day. He is tired at the end of each session with the physical therapist. He is progressing well with his treatment plan and will be released before the weekend.

EXERCISE 1-21 Use each of the verb phrases in a complete sentence. These are sample sentences only. Yours will vary.

1. will repeat

   The patient will repeat each exercise five times.

2. has diagnosed

   The doctor has diagnosed Bob's tumor to be benign.

3. has lost

   She has lost an appeal with the medical board.

4. will be removed

   The scar tissue will be removed later.

5. have felt

   We have felt the pain of losing a loved one.

EXERCISE 1-22 Finish the clauses to create an independent clause or sentence. These are sample sentences only. Yours will vary.

1. The patient will go home soon.
2. The tissue will regenerate new cells.
3. The phlebotomist handled the frightened child with patience and expertise.
4. Seeing the therapist will help you make an informed decision.
5. After the consultation, the nurse relaxed.

EXERCISE 1-23 Write a sentence that includes these subordinating conjunctions. These are sample sentences only. Yours will vary.

1. Because of the nature of his illness, the treatment options are limited.
2. Since she opted for laser surgery, her recovery time is less.
3. Until the doctor releases him, he may not check out of the hospital.
4. A person should seek medical attention whenever there is a question about a sudden change in health.
5. The nurse will dress the patient before her family arrives.

UNIT PROOFREADING EXERCISES

Read the passage below and make the corrections by crossing out the errors; then replace each error with the correction.

Ms. Robinswood wants to visit her doctor. Three ~~year~~ (years) ago she had three ~~sarcoma~~ (sarcomata or sarcomas) removed. She believes everyone should see ~~their~~ (his or her) doctor once a year. One of her friends agrees with ~~she~~ (her); however, most ~~don'~~ (don't.) They believe they are healthy. Ms. Robinswood is ~~caution~~ (cautious) about her health. Because she had cancer one ~~times~~ (time) before, she is more careful than her friends. She appears ~~health~~, (healthy), but she just wants make sure she is well.

UNIT REVISION EXERCISES

Read the sentences below and correct the form of the underlined word so that the correct form of the medical terminology is used in each sentence.

1. The gauze formed a protect layer. (protective)
2. The psychology will now see the patient. (psychologist)
3. She will excision the tumor. (excise)
4. Ambulation the patient this morning. (Ambulate)
5. The surgery was invade. (invasive)
6. The oncology will see new patients; she has expanded her practice. (oncologist)
7. Five patients had urinalysis completed by the laboratory technician this morning. (urinalyses)
8. Doctors' diagnosis sometimes vary, based on experience and training. (diagnoses)

Revise these sentences to make them complete sentences.

9. Because he is worried about recurrence.

   Because he is worried about recurrence of the cancer, he is careful to schedule his appointments with the oncologist and follow his care plan.

10. The consultation with Dr. Ishmel is important for you and I.

    The consultation with Dr. Ishmel is important for you and me.

UNIT 1 SELF-CHECK

Label each underlined word with its part of speech. Use adjective, adverb, conjunction, interjection, noun, pronoun, preposition, and verb.

noun 1. Atherosclerosis, a form of arteriosclerosis, is a degenerative vascular disorder.

verb 2. The specialist will call the patient as soon as the blood work is reviewed.

adjective 3. Lyme disease can be an undetected illness.

adverb 4. Mice suddenly lost weight when injected with leptin.

preposition 5. Inflammation is a main mechanism in heart disease.

conjunction 6. Because so many factors were involved in his treatment, a team of medical staff worked together to form a plan.

Underline the phrases in the sentence below.

7. Now the medical community has gained more knowledge about the complexity of this disease as a result of the research provided by the Centers for Disease Control.

Underline the main clause in each sentence below.

8. The condition of the patient is improving, which has made the family hopeful.

9. Because the drug is still in the experimental stage, it is unavailable to the general public.

10. Insects that carry parasites often infect people through vector sites.

UNIT 2: SENTENCE BASICS

EXERCISE 2-1 Indicate if the sentence is a complete sentence (CS) or a fragment (F)

1. F The doctor seems.
2. CS The workplace is stressful, so we need to have hobbies to relax.
3. F Because of the way that the man and woman argued in front of the nurses.
4. CS The diagnosis was made after many tests.
5. CS Consulting with one another was the medical team.
6. CS By caring for your eyesight, you will retain your excellent vision.
7. CS For me, I need reassurance that I will be healthy again.
8. CS The drugs are powerful.
9. CS Avoid the dangerous streets; stay home tonight.
10. F The patient with his leg in a cast.

EXERCISE 2-2 Underline the subject once and the verb twice.

1. Our relationship with food changes over time.
2. Many people now avoid trans fats in their diets.
3. Remember to relax. [You—understood subject]
4. Carbohydrates provide most of our calories.
5. In the average American diet, carbohydrates make up about 50% of our calories.
6. The secret to making good coffee is in the bean.
7. The doctor and nurses are in a staff meeting.
8. The patient must sign the medical release form.
9. Her condition is becoming progressively worse.
10. Your insurance card will be mailed to your home address.

EXERCISE 2-3 Write a simple sentence of your own with each of the following terms.

Refer to unit glossary for definitions of these words. These are sample sentences only. Yours will vary.

1. prenatal

   Prenatal care is critical for the health of the mother and her unborn baby.

2. salmonella

   Salmonella is a food-borne illness that can be fatal.

3. grievance

   His grievance was filed against the administrators of the long-term care center.

4. myalgia

   Myalgia is generalized muscle pain, and it is sometimes difficult to treat.

5. managed care

   Managed care is a trend that has gained popularity with Americans.

Exercise 2-4 Use these compound subjects and verbs in sentences of your own. These are sample sentences only. Yours will vary.

1. purchase and restock

   The pharmacy technican will purchase and restock the shelves in the drugstore.

2. Dr. Smith and Dr. Halle

   Dr. Smith and Dr. Halle share suite 302 in the Morris Building.

3. prescribed and filled

   The doctor prescribed and filled the medicine for the elderly homebound resident.

4. clean and suture

   The doctor will clean and suture the hand wound.

5. compare and sort

   The dental assistant will compare and sort the sample products that came in today.

Exercise 2-5 State whether each of the following sentences is a simple sentence (SS), a command (Com), a question (Qu), or an exclamatory sentence (Ex). Write the answer on the line provided.

Com **1.** Contact the hospice coordinator at (425) 555-0100.

Qu **2.** Is there an operating room available now?

Com **3.** Sign your legal name on this insurance form.

SS **4.** Esophagitis can be treated easily.

Qu **5.** Will this medication decrease my appetite?

Com **6.** Call the head nurse STAT!

Ex **7.** What a lovely day!

SS **8.** Your daughter is recovering quickly.

Qu **9.** When will the doctor sign the release papers?

Com **10.** Please remove your glasses.

EXERCISE 2-6 Write one sentence of your own in each type below. These are sample sentences only. Yours will vary.

1. simple sentence

   Nurses are in demand today.

2. command

   Open the elevator door, please.

3. question

   When will the doctor be in?

4. exclamatory sentence

   Help!

EXERCISE 2-7 Use each of the following strong verbs in a sentence of your own. Refer to the unit glossary for definitions of these words. These are sample sentences only. Yours will vary.

1. intubate

   The lab technician can intubate a patient quickly because of the job experience.

2. elicit

   Please elicit a response from Ms. Rogers.

3. palpate

   The doctor palpated the patient's abdominal cavity.

4. incubate

   The bacterial samples incubate in this protective environment.

5. ligate

   The nurse ligated the patient's arm in place to avoid further nerve damage.

UNIT PROOFREADING EXERCISES

Make the corrections by crossing out any errors or making edits by adding or removing words or punctuation.

> *A new medical devise has been approved by the Food and Drug Administration. Which is called The Merci Retriever. What device use? The device is made out of nitinol wire. Designed to rid the brain of blood clots. Blood clots debilitating and deadly.*

Rewrite this passage here:

This is one way to revise the passage. Your answer may vary.

> *A new medical <u>device, which is called the Merci Retriever,</u> has been approved by the Food and Drug Administration. What is the device used for? The device is made out of nitinol <u>wire, and it is designed</u> to rid the brain of blood clots. Blood clots <u>can be</u> debilitating and deadly.*

UNIT REVISION EXERCISES

Revise each sentence or sentence part to have a specific subject and a strong verb. You may need to add or remove words. Ensure that all sentences are complete.

1. There are plastic gloves to use for aseptic reasons.

   Use plastic gloves for aseptic reasons.

2. There are the autopsy results.

   The autopsy results reveal a massive stroke.

3. It is estimated that the doctor will arrive by 9 o'clock.

   The doctor arrives at 9 o'clock.

4. Call me sometime today.

   Call me at noon today.

5. She has pain.

   Her intense pain radiates from her chest cavity downward.

6. It is negative.

   Such sarcasm creates negative communication.

7. Cold compresses to the thigh.

   Apply cold compresses to the thigh.

8. If you stay fit.

   If you stay fit, your health will continue to improve.

9. There are too many guests in this room.

   The number of guests is limited to two in this room; please respect the hospital rules.

10. This stuff needs to be taken somewhere.

    The newspapers and magazines create clutter; please remove them.

UNIT 2 SELF-CHECK

Read each of the sentences below. Determine whether it is a independent clause (IC) or a dependent clause (DC).

IC **1.** When will the catheter be in place?

IC **2.** The technician prepared the slides for the supervisor to review.

DC **3.** If your asthma attack is triggered by cigarette smoke.

DC **4.** Because lowering your cholesterol may be difficult.

IC **5.** Your risk of a second stroke may be reduced by this medication.

Read each sentence below. Determine what essential sentence part is missing—subject (subj), verb (vb), or complete thought (ct)—or if the sentence is correct as written (ok). Write your answer on the line.

vb **6.** How we make healthcare coverage decisions.

ok **7.** Take antibiotics only as prescribed.

vb **8.** Many schools vision screening programs beginning in preschool years.

subj **9.** Also contribute to type 2 diabetes.

ok **10.** Eating healthfully and working out do not have to be difficult.

11–12. Read the boldfaced medical term and its definition. Then create a sentence of your own using this term.

edema: noun—a condition; an abnormal accumulation of fluids in the intercellular spaces of the body

Edema often appears around a patient's ankles.

throat culture: noun—a procedure; a bacteriological test used to identify throat pathogens, especially those associated with group A streptococci

The doctor will do a throat culture to make a diagnosis.

UNIT 3: EXPANDING SENTENCE BASICS

EXERCISE 3-1 Use this format to create appositive phrases of your own. Refer to the unit glossary for definitions of these words. Your answers should be close to these.

Noun being described	Comma	Modifying words (adjectives)	Noun/Pronoun	Comma
pediatrician	,	**a children's**	**doctor**	,
ringworm	,	**a parasitic**	**infection**	,
contusion	,	**a**	**bruise**	,
lipid	,	**a**	**fat**	,

EXERCISE 3-2 Write simple sentences that include an appositive phrase. Follow each word with an appositive phrase that describes or clarifies the term. Refer to the unit glossary for definitions of these words.

For example: oncologist

The oncologist, *a doctor specializing in treating cancers,* was well versed in a wide variety of treatment options.

I need to see the oncologist, *a doctor specializing in treating cancers.*

1. tumor

The doctor said that my cancer, a tumor, will be removed next week.

2. Braille

The series of bumps in patterns, Braille, allows the blind to read.

3. ethnicity

His ethnicity, American-born Chinese, has never been an issue for him.

4. chicken pox

Chicken pox, a virus, is contagious.

5. thrombosis

His leg has a clot, a thrombosis.

EXERCISE 3-3 Revise each sentence to include an appositive phrase. These are sample sentences only. Yours will vary.

1. Intimacy is the feeling of closeness with another person, and it is characterized by feelings of love, friendship, and companionship.

   Intimacy, the feeling of closeness with another person, is characterized by feelings of love, friendship, and companionship.

2. Medical asepsis refers to medical practices that reduce microorganisms and their transmission from one person to another and is referred to as clean technique.

   Medical asepsis, medical practices that reduce microorganisms and their transmission from one person to another, is referred to as clean technique.

3. Hand washing is central to isolation technique, and it is the single most important way to prevent the spread of infection.

   Hand washing, the single most important way to prevent the spread of infection, is central to isolation technique.

4. The physical therapist does not work Monday; the physical therapist is a part-time student.

   The physical therapist, a part-time student, does not work Monday.

5. Presbyopia is due to a loss of elasticity in the eye's crystalline lens. Presbyopia is known as farsightedness.

   Presbyopia, farsightedness, is due to a loss of elasticity in the eye's crystalline lens.

EXERCISE 3-4 Write compound sentences of your own in this pattern. These are sample sentences only. Yours will vary.

Independent Clause	,	Coordinating Conjunction	Independent Clause	.
Good health care is important	,	and	it is often expensive	.
Bob wants to lose weight	,	but	he does not want to diet and exercise	.
We will make a doctor's appointment	,	for (meaning: because)	this pain in my right side has continued for several days	.
He does not eat fresh fruit	,	nor	does he eat fresh vegetables	.
We can increase exercising	,	or	we can cut 500 calories from our diets	.
We need to visit the dentist	,	so	I will make an appointment	.
We want to be healthy	,	yet	we do not want to make life changes	.

EXERCISE 3-5 Write compound sentences of your own in this pattern. These are sample sentences only. Yours will vary.

Independent Clause	;	Conjunctive Adverb	,	Independent Clause	.
The doctor will examine the patient	;	therefore	,	the medical assistant will put the patient into an examination room	.
The child has a persistent cough	;	however	,	no fever is present	.
Avian flu is life threatening	;	nevertheless	,	people should take precaution but not become panicked	.
The course is 12 months	;	consequently	,	the state examination will take place next December	.
Prenatal care is vital to the mother and baby's health	;	therefore	,	Sally should schedule her first doctor's appointment now	.

EXERCISE 3-6 Write compound sentences of your own in this pattern. These are sample sentences only. Yours will vary.

Independent Clause	;	Independent Clause	.
Eating healthy foods is important	;	good nutrition depends on making good food choices.	.
Being a nurse requires specialized training	;	nurses need many people skills	.
Having a pet is comforting for senior citizens	;	pets bring the elderly a sense of security	.
Caring for others takes patience	;	the rewards are many	.

EXERCISE 3-7 The complex sentences below are partially written. Complete these complex sentences following the given pattern. These are sample sentences only. Yours will vary.

Dependent Clause	,	Independent Clause	.
When the flu season begins	,	get plenty of rest, wash your hands often, and drink extra fluids	
After the technician completes taking the X-rays	,	they will be read by a radiologist	.
Since Bob needed some advice about flossing	,	the dental assistant helped him	.
As the surgical technician prepared the instruments	,	the surgeon was scrubbing for the surgery	.
Although the patient did not want more tests	,	the doctor ordered a few more tests	.

EXERCISE 3-8 The complex sentences below are partially written. Complete these complex sentences following the given pattern. These are sample sentences only. Yours will vary.

Independent Clause	Dependent Clause	.
The pharmacist can answer your prescription questions	if you will wait for a few minutes	.
The patient was at ease	since the nurse seemed very helpful	.
Certified nursing assistants provide for the basic daily care of the residents	because they are the first line of care for the long-term facility's residents	.
She may stay in the hospital for another day	if more recovery time is needed	.
Hospice is an organization designed to assist family with the care of their terminally ill loved ones	that can be very helpful for family members	.

EXERCISE 3-9 The complex sentences below are partially written. Complete these complex sentences following the given pattern. These are sample sentences only. Yours will vary.

Independent Clause Starts	,	Dependent Clause	,	Independent Clause Ends	.
Some patients	,	who are allergic to many medicines	,	do not rely on medication	.
The medicine	,	which the doctor prescribed	,	changes the color of the patient's urine	.
Diabetes	,	which is more prevalent today	,	has two types, type 1 and type 2	.
Betty	,	who was treated by this physician	,	seems to be feeling a lot better	.

EXERCISE 3-10 Review the compound-complex sentence patterns. Write four sentences of your own using this sentence type. Use appropriate medical terminology and the context of health care for your subject matter. Refer to the unit glossary for possible words to use in your sentences. Your answers will vary.

1. The doctor was attending to the sick woman when his beeper went off; he was needed in room 206 immediately.
2. Answers Vary
3. Answers Vary
4. Answers Vary

EXERCISE 3-11 Shorten these sentences by making the clauses into phrases. These are sample sentences only. Yours will vary.

1. The presence of group A streptococci, which are bacteriological throat pathogens, needs to be confirmed.

   The presence of group A streptococci, bacteriological throat pathogens, needs to be confirmed.

2. Doctors who are called gerontologists diagnose and treat aging patients.

   Doctors, gerontologists, diagnose and treat aging patients.

3. A new device that is referred to as the Merci Retriever can remove blood clots from the brain.

   A new device, the Merci Retriever, can remove blood clots from the brain.

4. West Nile virus, which is a mosquito-borne virus, appears to be on the rise in the western portions of the United States.

   West Nile virus, a mosquito-borne virus, appears to be on the rise in the western portions of the United States.

EXERCISE 3-12 Underline the main idea in the sentences below. These are sample sentences only. Yours will vary.

1. When your doctor is off duty, other doctors are designated to provide for your care.
2. Healthcare agencies developed policies that describe the guidelines under which patients may read their records.
3. A law is an established and enforced rule of conduct that is intended to protect the rights of people.
4. An anecdotal note is a written record that presents the facts of a specific event.
5. Military time is a method of expressing time that uses a different four-digit number for each of the day's hours and minutes.

UNIT PROOFREADING EXERCISES

Read the paragraph below. Edit the sentences for correct sentence punctuation. Add or delete punctuation as needed.

> *Many young people are concerned about their body images. They do not want to be overweight [;] they do not want to be too tall or too short. Peer pressure is very strong during the adolescent period. Any change in a body ~~[,]~~ is noticed. Sometimes teens are teased[,] so they feel even more self-conscious. These issues about body image are reinforced by the media[,] which plays advertisements showing skinny bodies, lots of skin ~~[;]~~ [,] and a carefree lifestyle. It is easy to understand. Many youth feel ashamed by their changing bodies and weight gain. During this time[,] it is important that parents ensure a proper diet, plenty of exercise, and positive mentoring of friends and family.*

UNIT REVISION EXERCISES

Change these clauses into appositive phrases. These are sample sentences only. Yours will vary.

1. The surgeon, who is a pediatric dermatologist, suggested that we wait until Brittany is past her growth spurts before we attempt surgery.

   The surgeon, a pediatric dermatologist, suggested that we wait until Brittany is past her growth spurts before we attempt surgery.

2. The medicine, which is called Bactrim Suspension, is commonly used for ear infections in children.

   The medicine, Bactrim Suspension, is commonly used for ear infections in children.

3. The practice moved to a new building, which is called the Highway Medical Center.

   The practice moved to a new building, the Highway Medical Center.

4. Some herbal remedies, which may be popular but untested medicines, can be dangerous if the dosing is not controlled.

   Some herbal remedies, popular but untested medicines, can be dangerous if the dosing is not controlled.

5. Brown rice, which is a high-fiber food, is popular with many people who are watching their intake of carbohydrates.

   Brown rice, a high-fiber food, is popular with many people who are watching their intake of carbohydrates.

Make these compound-complex sentences into two shorter sentences.

6. The budget needs to cover needed equipment; the medical staff believes that a new autoclave will ensure instrument sterilization in a shorter amount of time and at a lower cost.

   The budget needs to cover needed equipment. The medical staff believes that a new autoclave will ensure instrument sterilization in a shorter amount of time and at a lower cost.

7. The medicine cart that needs to be repaired is missing a wheel part, so the cart always travels at an angle instead of in a straight line.

   The medicine cart that needs to be repaired is missing a wheel part. The cart always travels at an angle instead of in a straight line.

8. The floor volunteers have done a nice job of ensuring that patients have reading materials; in addition, they are providing opportunities for light discussion, which is so important for those patients who have been in the hospital a long time.

   The floor volunteers have done a nice job of ensuring that patients have reading materials. They are providing opportunities for light discussion, which is so important for those patients who have been in the hospital a long time.

UNIT 3 SELF-CHECK

Use the sentences to create a new sentence in the pattern requested. These are sample sentences only. Yours will vary.

1. The doctor specializes in pediatric brain surgeries. The doctor is a pediatric neurologist. (Combine to form a simple sentence that includes an appositive phrase.)

   The doctor, a pediatric neurologist, specializes in pediatric brain surgeries.

2. People are living longer. Blood pressure tends to rise with age. It also rises with weight gain or obesity. (Combine to form a compound sentence that is joined with *and.*)

   People are living longer, and blood pressure tends to rise with age, and it also rises with weight gain or obesity.

3. A new test for cholesterol is being researched. This test allows the blood to be tested any time. The current test requires the patient fast for 12 hours prior to the test. (Combine to form a compound-complex sentence.)

   A new test for cholesterol is being researched; this test allows the blood to be tested any time, while the current test requires the patient fast for 12 hours prior to the test.

4. Research has shown a link between soft drinks and type 2 diabetes. We need to encourage alternatives to sugary beverages for our children. (Combine to form a complex sentence.)

   Because research has shown a link between soft drinks and type 2 diabetes, we need to encourage alternatives to sugary beverages for our children.

Choose from these categories to label each sentence or sentence part below.

Appositive phrase	Fragment
Coordinating conjunction	Simple sentence
Conjunctive adverb	Compound sentence
Subordinating conjunction	Complex sentence

5. Conjunctive adverb ; therefore,
6. Simple sentence The call for type O blood has been placed.
7. Subordinating conjunction although
8. Compound sentence The pharmacy is about to close; the pharmacist will still assist you.
9. Fragment Since the beginning of the clinic construction
10. Appositive phrase , a registered nurse,
11. Coordinating conjunction or
12. Complex sentence While the baby is resting, you need to call your insurance provider.

UNIT 4: EFFECTIVE SENTENCE STRUCTURES

EXERCISE 4-1 Read the sentences below and indicate the whether each is written in the active or passive voice.

Sentences for Review	Voice of Verb: Active or Passive
The new procedure is being reviewed by the hospital board.	passive
Nurses attended a training session in the conference room.	active
A mistake was made in the documentation of this case.	passive
The reference manuals were placed in the staff work room.	passive
The certified nursing assistants assisted the nursing staff at the healthcare fair.	active

EXERCISE 4-2 Provide the active voice for each of the sentences below. These are sample sentences only. Yours will vary.

Sentence Written in Passive Voice	Revision in Active Voice
The nurse was assigned a new shift.	The supervisor assigned the nurse to a new shift.
The outdated medical records were shredded.	The clerk shredded the outdated medical records.

The extraction was done in the dentist's office.	The dentist extracted the tooth in his office.
The bandage was removed and discarded.	The nurse removed and discarded the bandage.
Blood pressure readings were taken twice a day.	The patient took his blood pressure twice a day.

EXERCISE 4-3 Make the revision to rid the sentence of ineffective starters. These are sample sentences only. Yours will vary.

Ineffective Sentence Starters	Revised Sentence Starters
There were last-minute arrangements that needed to be made prior to patient's admission to the residential center.	Last-minute arrangements needed to be made prior to made to patient's admission to the residential center.
It is necessary for some medical staff to have beepers in this wing of the hospital.	Some medical staff need to have beepers in this wing of the hospital.
There is a requirement that you submit to a urinalysis for drug testing prior to employment.	You must submit to a urinalysis for drug testing prior to employment
It is our mission to serve all patients who request medical care and family counseling.	Our mission is to serve all patients who request medical care and family counseling.
It is advised that the patient should not participate in vigorous activity.	The patient should not participate in vigorous activity.

EXERCISE 4-4 Write one sentence for each pattern given below. These are sample sentences only. Yours will vary.

Rules for Commas with Clauses	Examples
Use a comma followed by a coordinating conjunction *(and, but, for, or, nor, yet, so)* to separate two main clauses.	The pain continues, so I will see the doctor today.
Use a comma to separate an initial dependent clause from an independent clause.	Because the tooth is loose, I anticipate it will fall out soon.
Use a comma before a clause that begins with *which. Which* introduces a clause that provides extra information, so it is separated by one or more commas depending on its location in a sentence.	This is the hospital, which has a reputation of excellent care for stroke patients.

EXERCISE 4-5 Write one sentence for each pattern given below. These are sample sentences only. Yours will vary.

Rules for Commas with Words and Phrases	Examples
Use a comma for a series	We need to take your temperature, get your current weight, and check your blood pressure.
Use a comma after introductory comments such as *Well, Oh, Yes, No*, etc.	Well, I am not sure. Let me ask the doctor.
Use a comma after introductory phrases.	Because of his illness, we are not to leave town.
Use a comma between multiple adjectives before a noun.	The red, sore, enlarged tonsils are infected.
Use a comma after a person's name and before the title	Billie White, MD, will see new patients again in January.
Use commas around appositive phrases if they are mid-sentence and before a final appositive phrase in a sentence.	The doctor, a gynecologist, has a new practice.

EXERCISE 4-6 Write one sentence for each pattern given below. These are sample sentences only. Yours will vary.

Rules for Using Semicolons	Examples
Use a semicolon to separate two independent clauses.	The patient needs immediate care; please ask the doctor to come to room 230 stat.
Use a semicolon with a conjunctive adverb and a comma to separate two independent clauses.	The man is losing his sight; therefore, he may no longer drive.
Use a semicolon to separate items in a series that has internal commas.	We have medical centers in Seattle, Washington; Los Angeles, California; and Orlando, Florida.

EXERCISE 4-7 Write one sentence for each pattern given below. These are sample sentences only. Yours will vary.

Rules for Using Colons	Examples
Use a colon preceding a list or series that is not introduced by a verb.	Our assistant will purchase these office supplies: large paper clips, copy paper, pens, notepads, and envelopes.
Use a colon to distinguish hours from minutes in time.	The surgery is scheduled for 8:00 in the morning.
Use a colon after a formal salutation in a business letter.	Dear Doctor Bryan Booth:
Use a colon to emphasize a word, phrase, clause, or sentence that explains or adds impact to the main clause.	Individuals can make practical decisions about their health: They can make regular dental appointments and brush and floss daily.
Use a colon to distinguish between a title, subtitle, volume and page, and chapter and verse.	In the reference guide section 1:09, you will find a discussion about preventive care.
Use a colon to introduce a quotation, question, or sentence.	The doctor inquired to the family: "When did the patient decide to call hospice instead of continuing treatment?"

EXERCISE 4-8 Write one sentence for each pattern given below.

Rules for Using Hyphens	Examples
Use a hyphen for compound adjectives that modify one word, such as family-oriented practice, one-way street, one-in-ten chance.	Shaken-baby syndrome is often seen in abused infants and children.
Use a hyphen for writing out compound numbers between 21 and 99, such as twenty-one or fifty-five.	This is the twenty-fifth procedure this week.
Use a hyphen with fractions, such as two-thirds or one-fourth.	One-third of our staff speaks a second language.
Use a hyphen to join certain prefixes and roots such as *self-*, *all-*, and *ex-*. Refer to a dictionary if unsure.	Self-care is a skill that this office promotes.
Use a hyphen to divide a word at its syllable division point at the end of a line.	All of our staff must possess the communication skills con-sistent with the philosophy of the doctors who own this business.

EXERCISE 4-9 Revise each sentence providing effective vocabulary.

Examples of Ineffective Vocabulary	Revisions
The man is all scratched up.	The man has lesions and abrasions on his forearms.
The knife wound butchered him like a chicken on the cutting block.	The knife wounds left deep lacerations.

I am happy.	I feel content with my career decisions.
I believe that she feels sad about the death of her mama.	Maggie feels depressed by her mother's death.
She has a big black splotch on her leg.	She has a dark lesion on her leg.

UNIT PROOFREADING EXERCISES

Read the following passage. Then neatly cross out the errors and make the changes necessary for clear communication.

> *~~Sumamry of the Patient's Writes~~*
>
> *Summary of Patients' Rights*
>
> *The ~~american hospital association~~ published The Patient's Bill of Rights in 1973. In my opinion,*
> *American Hospital Association*
> *the purpose of this document focuses on the ~~responsible~~ of the hospitals and the patients. The objective is to*
> *responsibilities*
> *increase communication and collaboration between these parties. The patient is supposed to get consideration*
> *and respect while receiving care ~~[;]~~ true and ~~under standable~~ information about his or her condition, privacy,*
> *, understandable*
> *and confidentiality and a response to treatment request. The patient's responsibilities include giving up any*
> *information that might ~~effect~~ his or her treatment, insurance information, and pertinent lifestyle information.*
> *affect*
> *The goal is to ensure that both the hospital and the patient get the necessary information to provide and receive the best care possible.*

UNIT REVISION EXERCISES

Revise these sentences to ensure more specific expression. These are sample sentences only. Yours will vary.

1. For this procedure, there are eight steps that must be carried out.

For this procedure, eight steps must be carried out.

2. It is assumed that this individual is a hypochondriac.

This individual is a hypochondriac.

3. There is a dental assistant who tells everybody how important brushing and flossing are to do.

A dental assistant tells the patients how important brushing and flossing are.

Revise the following sentences to include semicolons, colons, commas, and hyphens.

4. The patient needs to ingest fat soluble vitamins.

The patient needs to ingest fat-soluble vitamins.

5. The autonomic system has two divisions the sympathetic and the parasympathetic.

The autonomic system has two divisions, the sympathetic and the parasympathetic.

6. Fellow healthcare professionals tonight my talk will cover breast research.

Fellow health care professionals, tonight my talk will cover breast research.

7. An injured man came into the emergency entrance; his wound was v shaped.

   An injured man came into the emergency entrance; his wound was v-shaped.

8. The diet was rich in calcium potassium minerals and folic acid.

   The diet was rich in calcium, potassium, minerals, and folic acid.

9. Dietitians are hired to ensure proper and restorative nutritional intake long term care residents need someone to assist them to ensure they have a balanced diet.

   Dietitians are hired to ensure proper and restorative nutritional intake; long-term care residents need someone to assist them to ensure they have a balanced diet.

Change this sentence from passive to active.

10. The surgical procedure was completed with the use of a tiny laser.

    The surgeon used a tiny laser to complete the surgical procedure.

UNIT 4 SELF-CHECK

Mark the sentences as correct or rewrite, making the changes as needed.

1. *Three categories of community agencies exist to provide numerous patient services; private, governmental, and nonprofit.*

   Three categories of community agencies exist to provide numerous patient services: private, governmental, and nonprofit.

2. *The seven-teen page document belongs to Dr. Fields.*

   The seventeen-page document belongs to Dr. Fields.

3. *He is part of a family oriented dental practice.*

   He is part of a family-oriented dental practice.

4. *The plan is to operate however if the tests come back with new information that plan can change.*

   The plan is to operate; however, if the tests come back with new information, that plan can change.

Rewrite as active sentences.

5. *The doctor was asked to explain his decision to the committee.*

   The committee asked the doctor to explain his decision.

6. *The old fabric chairs in the sun room were recycled.*

   Theresa recycled the old fabric chairs in the sun room.

7. *The excision was done in outpatient surgery wing of the hospital.*

   The surgeon performed the excision in the outpatient surgery wing of the hospital.

8. *The tumor was removed and sent to the lab.*

   The surgeon removed the tumor and sent it to the lab.

Revise each sentence to ensure effective communication.

9. *I think that the kid was all banged up.*

   The child had contusions and lacerations all over his body.

10. *It is my opinion that the insurance is the best thing since sliced bread.*

   Insurance is the best policy for ensuring equal access to professional care.

Look at the medical terminology in boldface below. Write a sentence of your own using the terms.

lymphoidectomy (*noun*) surgical removal of lymphoid tissue

11. Dr. Doyle performed the lymphoidectomy last Friday.

incise (*verb*) to make a cut into; to cut with a sharp instrument

12. He will incise the vein to remove the clot.

UNIT 5: COMMON SENTENCE ERRORS

EXERCISE 5-1 Write *S* for singular or *P* for plural in the blank to the right of each word or word group.

1. phlebotomist ___S___
2. a doctor who ___S___
3. any kind ___S___
4. somebody ___S___
5. Sal, along with the boys ___S___
6. all of the staff ___P___
7. ten pounds ___S___ (seen as one amount)
8. a few thermometers ___S___
9. therapy ___S___
10. bacterium ___S___

EXERCISE 5-2 Underline the verb that agrees with the subject.

1. Economics (do, does) influence health care decisions.
2. There (is, are) no staff member available to assist the patient.
3. Either the parent or the guardian (need, needs) to authorize this procedure.
4. Training and experience (contribute, contributes) to the excellence of Bella Hospital.
5. Each of you (have, has) a task to accomplish in Room 523.

6. Without computers, the medical receptionists (<u>do</u>, does) not have access to your insurance records.
7. The medical team (<u>is</u>, are) waiting for the lab results.
8. In the newborn area, registered nurses (<u>gather</u>, gathers) to view the twins.
9. Neither the child nor the parents (was, <u>were</u>) feeling well.
10. The doctor, along with his assistants, (intend, <u>intends</u>) to operate to remove the tumor.

Exercise 5-3 Complete the sentences below. These are sample sentences only. Yours will vary.

1. Either the patients or the nurse <u>wants to talk to the doctor.</u>
2. The staff <u>gathered for the meeting.</u>
3. Every one of the <u>residents has an interview with the director of nursing.</u>
4. The nurse, together with the medical assistants, <u>is working with the patients' families to provide optimal care.</u>
5. Dental assistants and dental hygienists <u>promote dental hygiene.</u>

Exercise 5-4 Write the pronoun in the blank to the right of each word or word group.

1. phlebotomist <u>he or she</u>
2. Mr. Edward Smithers <u>he</u>
3. anyone <u>he or she</u>
4. somebody <u>he or she</u>
5. Sally, along with the boys <u>she</u>
6. all of the instruments <u>they</u>
7. ten pounds <u>it</u> (seen as an amount)
8. a few thermometers <u>they</u>
9. therapy <u>it</u>
10. specimen slides <u>they</u>

Exercise 5-5 Underline the pronoun that agrees with its antecedent.

1. The cost of care may make a person decide (<u>he</u>, they) cannot afford the elective surgery.
2. Each of the female patients needs to have (<u>her</u>, their) own prenatal file.
3. Either the parent or the guardian needs to authorize this claim for (<u>his,</u> their) child.
4. Training is important for all new employees; (he, it, <u>they</u>) need to understand our policies and procedures.
5. How does the hospital handle (his, <u>its</u>) patients?
6. The administrator asked all of (we, <u>us</u>) to outline solutions to assist in the conflict resolution.
7. The medical laboratory is fully staffed; (their, <u>its</u>) employees are now in training.
8. The decision about elective care is between (he and she, <u>him and her</u>).

9. Neither the child nor the parents want (his, their) files reviewed.

10. The doctor, along with his assistants, will operate on (his, their) patient.

EXERCISE 5-6 Complete each sentence to include a pronoun that refers to an antecedent. Proofread to ensure the pronoun agrees with its antecedent. These are sample sentences only. Yours will vary.

1. Neither the patient nor the doctor is sure of the cause of the infection.
2. How do the staff use their professional development hours?
3. Each patient has a right to appeal his medical bills.
4. The clinic is open 285 days of the year.
5. Two patients refuse to take their medications during her shift.

EXERCISE 5-7 Read the sentences and place a check in front of those sentences that have a dangling modifier.

√ 1. Having completed the assignment, the list was reviewed by the certified nursing assistant.

_ 2. Calling the patient's family, the nurse was delighted with the patient's condition.

√ 3. The bandage by pouring warm water over the incision site was removed by the nurse.

√ 4. After completing multiple tests, the report was sent to the doctor by the laboratory assistant.

√ 5. Lacking O positive blood, the patient's surgery was delayed.

EXERCISE 5-8 Revise the sentences to remove the dangling modifiers. These are sample sentences only. Yours will vary.

1. After reading the article about Paxil, the information was helpful to the patient.

   After reading the article about Paxil, the patient found the information was helpful.

2. The chart, recovering from the procedure, is placed at the foot of the patient's bed.

   The chart is placed at the foot of the bed of the patient recovering from the procedure.

3. Hanging the IV, the pole needed to be stabilized by the nurse.

   Hanging the IV, the nurse stabilized the pole.

4. The medical receptionist compiled a letter, drafting the complaint to the insurance company.

   The medical receptionist, drafting the complaint to the insurance company, compiled a well-written letter filled with data.

5. The diagnosis refusing to believe the doctor upset the family.

   The diagnosis upset the family, who then refused to believe the doctor.

6. Eating the balanced diet, the nutritious foods took on a new meaning for the young diabetics.

   Eating the balanced diet, young diabetics need the nutritious foods to remain healthy.

7. Twisting the patient in a variety of positions, the muscles were viewed in a variety of positions by the physical therapists.

   The physical therapists, twisting the patient in a variety of positions, manipulated the patient's muscles in attempt to relieve pain.

8. Scanning the lumbar region, the MRI was used by the technician to locate the growth.

   Scanning the lumbar region, the technician used MRI to locate the growth.

9. Flossing daily, the teeth and gums are cleaned below the gum line.

   Flossing daily, the hygienist cleaned the teeth below the gum line.

10. Massaging the swollen area, the pain slowly dissipated.

    Massaging the swollen area, the therapist knew the pain would slowly dissipate.

EXERCISE 5-9 Underline the parallel structures in these sentences. These are sample sentences only. Yours will vary.

1. The patient has the right to know his prognosis and the need to know the medical implications.
2. In the morning and in the afternoon, the shift reports are conducted in Room 125.
3. The refusal to take the medicine and the desire to return home were her most common subjects of discussion.
4. The patient is stable and mobile.
5. The rehabilitation assistant ambulated the patient and then massaged the patient's legs after the walk this morning.
6. Removing the gauze and cleaning the wound, the nurse described the steps and showed the patient the method of wound care.
7. Changing colostomy bags takes skill and requires patience with new patients.
8. When the patient is angry and frustrated, the caregiver reminds the patient of his need to be motivated.
9. Human emotions and human behavior tell a great deal about the health of a patient.
10. Common sense and problem-solving logic can help a young mother determine when to call the doctor and when to wait before calling the doctor.

EXERCISE 5-10 Correct the errors in parallel structure in these sentences. These are sample sentences only. Yours will vary.

1. He wants to have peace of mind and avoidance of stress.

   He wants to have peace of mind and to avoid stress.

2. The nurse wanted to speak with the parents and told them about the therapy session.

   The nurse wanted to speak with the parents and to tell them about the therapy session.

3. The physician's assistant was tired, cold, and wanted to eat something.

   The physician's assistant was tired, cold, and hungry.

4. The supervisor tried to be helpful, encouraged and supporting of his team.

   The supervisor tried to be helpful and supportive of his team.

5. In an exhaustive search and reading lots of medical journals, the information about the procedure was found.

   In an exhaustive search and through medical journal reading, the information about the procedure was found.

6. The lack of personal care and of resources left the patient in poor condition before the surgery.

   The lack of personal care and absence of resources left the patient in poor condition before the surgery.

7. The doctor told the patient to schedule a follow-up appointment, but the patient decides that another visit is not necessary.

   The doctor told the patient to schedule a follow-up appointment, but the patient decided that another visit was not necessary.

8. The patient was uncomfortable and dissatisfaction with the care he was given.

   The patient was uncomfortable and dissatisfied with the care he was given.

9. The treatment options were discussed with the patient and her family; the decision is made a week ago to begin chemotherapy.

   The treatment options were discussed with the patient and her family; the decision was made a week ago to begin chemotherapy.

10. The clerical staff type, copy, file, and then need to mail their daily work.

    The clerical staff type, copy, file, and mail their daily work.

EXERCISE 5-11 Read the following sentences. If a shift in tense or an incorrect use of tense occurs, place an *X* on the blank by the sentence.

X **1.** The physician saw patients between 7:00 A.M. and 9:30 A.M. six days a week.

X **2.** When I need to see the dentist, I went to the closest one to my home.

X **3.** The patient was already prepared for the procedure; it will begin in about three minutes.

_ **4.** The surgery proceeded as planned and scheduled.

X **5.** Our office closes next April for a remodeling project.

EXERCISE 5-12 Use each term in a present-tense sentence. These are sample sentences only. Yours will vary.

1. bathe — We bathe the patients each day.
2. suture — The doctor sutures the wound in a *Z* pattern.
3. massage — The therapist massages the patient in an attempt to relax her.
4. bandage — Nurses bandage many wounds.
5. test — The students test all the time.

EXERCISE 5-13 Use each term in a past-tense sentence. These are sample sentences only. Yours will vary.

1. examine — The doctor examined my foot during the examination.
2. remove — The nursing assistant removed his gown carefully.
3. swipe — He swiped the insurance card through the machine.
4. excise — The surgeon excised the tumor.
5. trim — The dietitian trimmed the total amount of fat in daily intake.

EXERCISE 5-14 Use each term in a present-perfect sentence. These are sample sentences only. Yours will vary.

1. input The staff has input many ideas for the new medical wing.
2. inspire The medical team has inspired many students to achieve their goals.
3. make The nurse had made many beds today.
4. eat The patient has eaten his meal this morning.
5. clip The aide has clipped his nails once before.

UNIT PROOFREADING EXERCISES

Read the following paragraph and correct any errors in subject–verb agreement, pronoun–antecedent agreement, verb tense, dangling modifiers, parallel structure, and grammar.

Burns have been classified as first, second, or third degree depending on ~~its~~ (their) depth, not how much pain or damage has been done. A first-degree burn ~~reached~~ (reaches) the outer layer of skin. In this case, the skin ~~appear~~ (appears) dry, painful, and sensitive to touch (;) a sunburn ~~was~~ (is) an example of a first-degree burn. A second-degree burn ~~has damaged~~ (damages) several layers of skin. The skin ~~may became swell~~ (becomes swollen), puffy, weeping, or blistered. One example of a second-degree burn ~~might be~~ (is) a hot-water burn. A third-degree burn, ~~involved~~ (involving) all layers of the skin and any underlying tissue and/or organs, ~~has resulted~~ (results) in dry, pale white or charred black, swollen skin. Damaging or destroying the ~~nerve~~ (nerves), the (burn may cause the) patient ~~may experience~~ no or little pain. Third-degree burns need immediate medical attention.

UNIT REVISION EXERCISES

Each sentence below has one error in verb or pronoun usage or structure. Locate each error and revise the sentence. These are sample sentences only. Yours will vary.

1. Every one of the patients in this section of the wing need to receive his medication.

   Every one of the patients in this section of the wing needs to receive his medication.

2. Either of the drugs are used to treat this condition.

   Either of the drugs is used to treat this condition.

3. Not only is the doctor working in the hospital but in the residential community clinic too.

   Not only is the doctor working in the hospital, but he also is working in the residential community clinic too.

4. The patient needs to be bathed and attending the physical therapy session scheduled for 9:30 A.M.

   The patient needs to be bathed and taken to the physical therapy session scheduled for 9:30 A.M.

5. Microbiology was the scientific study of microorganisms.

   Microbiology is the scientific study of microorganisms.

UNIT 5 SELF-CHECK

1. Explain what a dangling modifier is. Why is a dangling modifier an error in sentence structure?

A dangling modifier is a group of words that are misplaced because this group does not modify the intended word. These often occur at the beginning of the sentence; however, a dangling modifier can occur elsewhere in the sentence. The error has to do with the structure and placement of the phrase in the sentence, not the form or grammar itself.

Read the sentences below. If the sentence is correct, mark *C* on the line. If it is incorrect, mark *W* on the line, then make the corrections in the sentence.

W 2. Each of the phlebotomists ~~complete~~ (completes) 100 blood draws this morning.

W 3. The cryoprobe is a device that ~~apply~~ (applies) cold to tissue.

W 4. Eating a diet rich in fruits and vegetables ~~are~~ (is) healthy and nutritious.

W 5. Sixty pounds ~~are~~ (is) a lot of weight to lose.

C 6. That safety harness is too loose.

C 7. Surgical instruments and equipment must be properly sterilized.

W 8. Infusion ~~are~~ (is) one of the methods of dispensing medications.

W 9. Pediatric patients need to feel secure, loved, and ~~being nurtured~~ (nurtured).

W 10. One of the keloids ~~are~~ (is) growing rapidly.

W 11. Economics ~~are~~ (is) involved in our decision to keep our insurance provider.

W 12. The doctor, along with his staff members, ~~report~~ (reports) to the hospital board.

UNIT 6: ACHIEVING MORE IN SENTENCE VARIETY

EXERCISE 6-1 Underline each gerund in the following sentences.

1. Talking to his visitors is how the patient spent his afternoon.
2. The radiologist appears to be reviewing the X-rays.
3. The residents of the long-term care facility enjoy talking with their doctors.
4. Working in a medical office is her preference.
5. By studying medical terminology, the clerks are more efficient in reviewing medical reports and documents.

EXERCISE 6-2 Complete these sentences that have gerunds in them. These are sample sentences only. Yours will vary.

1. Wiping the edges of the wound requires patience.
2. By seeing the film, the allied health students were enthused about patient care.
3. Giving a patient a bed bath helps the patient feel better.

4. By not eating, the patient had lost a lot of weight.

5. Transferring patients takes trained personnel who are familiar with transfer techniques.

EXERCISE 6-3 Draft sentences with the following verbs as gerunds and use these gerunds in the specified format. These are sample sentences only. Yours will vary.

1. diagnose Diagnosing lymphoma is done through a variety of tests.
2. massage Massaging the temples can alleviate a headache.
3. refer By referring to the Drug Guide, the students learned the top 50 medications.
4. prescribe The doctor has the duty of prescribing the medication.
5. input The technician finds inputting the data to be interesting.

EXERCISE 6-4 Revise the sentences below to include a gerund. You may need to rephrase parts of the sentences; however, attempt to maintain a similar meaning. These are sample sentences only. Yours will vary.

1. The promotion of a patient's independence is critical in assisting him to meet his healthcare needs.

   Promoting a patient's independence is critical in assisting him to meet his healthcare needs.

2. It is important to try to understand a patient's cultural background, for it allows healthcare professionals to understand the person's behavior.

   Understanding a patient's cultural background allows healthcare professionals to understand the person's behavior.

3. The plan for job duties and responsibilities for the new position should alleviate stress among the staff.

   Planning for job duties and responsibilities for the new position should alleviate stress among the staff.

4. It is important to identify alternatives for treatments for all patients, and it is part of his job.

   Identifying alternatives for treatments for all patients is part of his job.

5. The direction of information is the job of the center's administrator.

   Directing information is the job of the center's administrator.

6. In order to avoid legal suits, nursing staff should be knowledgeable of the patient's rights.

   Knowing the patient's rights can help nursing staff avoid lawsuits.

7. To care for the elderly takes a special person.

   Caring for the elderly takes a special person.

8. We hope to locate her closest relative, which may be difficult.

   Locating her closest relative may be difficult.

9. We expanded our diagnostic procedures to cover the national guidelines.

   Expanding our diagnostic procedures allows us to cover the national guidelines.

10. To wash one's hands is important to prevent the transfer of bacteria.

    Washing one's hands is important in preventing the transfer of bacteria.

EXERCISE 6-5 Underline each infinitive in the following sentences.

1. To review the screenings is her job.
2. The doctor to see is your primary care physician.
3. He wants to speak with his urologist sometime today.
4. The reason to be concerned is the rapid deterioration of the skin.
5. The doctor will call to schedule the lab work.

EXERCISE 6-6 Label the infinitive by function: noun, adjective, or adverb.

1. adjective The tooth to be filled is a molar.
2. noun To schedule the appointment, call the office after 8:00 A.M.
3. adjective The MRI to be taken is scheduled for Monday at 9:00 A.M.
4. noun The doctor asked the patient to call his office in two days.
5. adverb The nurses saved their money to have a party for the interns.
6. noun To be allowed to go home early required the patient's family to be available to assist him.
7. noun We wish to travel as VISTA nurses.
8. adjective Our collaborative efforts to give support aided in the patient's recovery.
9. adverb We advised him to seek treatment as soon as possible.
10. noun To have empathy is a workplace skill.

EXERCISE 6-7 Complete these sentences that have infinitives in them. These are sample sentences only. Yours will vary.

1. To relieve muscle tension is the purpose of the massage.
2. To inform your supervisor is critical in this incident.
3. Bob was unwilling to improve his position.
4. The nurses wished to study for their master's degree in nursing.
5. The reason to be concerned is your long-term health.

EXERCISE 6-8 Draft sentences using the following verbs as infinitives in the specified format. These are sample sentences only. Yours will vary.

1. diagnose To diagnose some illnesses requires many tests.
2. transport To transport the patient will require a hoist.
3. divide They want to divide the workload.
4. cure To cure cancer is our hope.
5. inject To inject the dye takes a skilled doctor.

Exercise 6-9 Revise the sentences below to include an infinitive. You may need to rephrase parts of the sentences; however, attempt to maintain a similar meaning. These are sample sentences only. Yours will vary.

1. The two clavicles help by bracing the shoulders and prevent forward motion.

   The two clavicles help to brace the shoulders and to prevent forward motion.

2. The medical assistant kept busy by calling patients reminding them of their upcoming appointments.

   The medical assistant kept busy by calling patients to remind them of their upcoming appointments.

3. Lifting properly prevents back injuries.

   To prevent back injuries, lift properly.

4. The nurse will be reviewing the patient care plan as part of her duties.

   To review the patient care plan is part of a nurse's duties.

5. The dentist is thinking about requesting the dental assistants be available for attending an after-work meeting.

   The dentist is thinking about requesting the dental assistants be available to attend an after-work meeting.

6. Warming up is important before exercising vigorously.

   To warm up is important before exercising vigorously.

7. Requesting that patients complete the health survey is part of our quality-assurance plan.

   To request that patients complete the health survey is part of our quality-assurance plan.

8. Discussing confidential information in the staff room is strictly against policy.

   To discuss confidential information in the staff room is strictly against policy.

9. Writing thank-you notes to the community volunteers is important.

   To write thank-you notes to the community volunteers is important.

10. Having your name removed from our mailing list is a quick procedure.

    To have your name removed from our mailing list is a quick procedure.

Exercise 6-10 Identify the participial phrases in the sentences.

1. Working as a medical assistant, she is content.
2. The patient, having lived alone for years, is having a difficult time adjusting to the group home.
3. Handing out the magazines, the volunteers provide a friendly face for the patients.
4. The wheelchair, broken and without a battery, needs to go to the repair center.
5. Removing his contacts, the patient is ready for the eyedrops.

Exercise 6-11 Complete these sentences that contain participial phrases. These are sample sentences only. Yours will vary.

1. Hugging her mother in the recovery room, the little girl was relieved.
2. Removing the gauze, the nurse saw the wound was healing.

3. Rubbing the patient's back, the therapist put the patient at ease.
4. The nurse, asking the visitors to wait outside the room, changed the patient's bandage.
5. Covering the patient with a drape, the medical assistant ensured patient privacy.
6. The doctor, speaking in a quiet voice, calmed Mrs. Williams.
7. The dental hygienist, wanting to ensure a proper exam, reread the patient's chart.
8. The ophthalmic assistant, handing the wand to the patient, explained the eye exam.
9. The medical team, wanting the patient to recover quickly, met with the patient and family about their rehabilitation program.
10. The allied health instructor, repeating the critical information, hinted that this information might be on an exam.

EXERCISE 6-12 Draft sentences with the following verbs as participles in the specified format. These are sample sentences only. Yours will vary.

1. diagnose — After diagnosing the woman's illness, the doctor met with her about treatment options.
2. transport — Transporting a patient, the nurse's aide moved slowly and carefully.
3. divide — Dividing the workload, the team was working well together.
4. cure — The doctor, curing the patient's parasitic infection, ensured that the patient understood that the skin lesions were permanent.
5. inject — Injecting the drug into the arm of the soldier, the doctor explained that there might be some swelling.

EXERCISE 6-13 Revise the sentences below to include a participle. You may need to rephrase parts of the sentences; however, attempt to maintain a similar meaning. These are sample sentences only. Yours will vary.

1. The patient, who refused to believe the test results, sought a second opinion.

   The patient, refusing to believe the test results, sought a second opinion.

2. The student was unable to remember the car accident; he led police to believe that he wasn't driving.

   Unable to remember the car accident, the student led police to believe that he wasn't driving.

3. The family members will learn to cope with his death, and they continue their pursuit of cancer research.

   Learning to cope with his death, the family will continue their pursuit of cancer research.

4. A nurse should possess the ability to educate the patient for self-care and health maintenance.

   Possessing the ability to educate the patient for self-care and health maintenance, the nurse plays a vital role.

5. It is important for a patient to understand the health–illness continuum because it shows that there is no specific point of wellness or illness.

   Understanding the health–illness continuum, the patient is able to learn that there is no specific point of wellness or illness.

6. Pediatricians encourage mothers to teach their children the importance of wearing seat belts, for it saves lives.

   Pediatricians, encouraging mothers to teach their children the importance of wearing seat belts, save lives.

7. The eye-care profession hopes to create optimal vision for the patients. The sophisticated measurement devices are used.

   By using the sophisticated measurement devices, the eye-care profession hopes to create optimal vision for the patients.

8. Eyeglass prescriptions always have a spherical power. These powers are calculated by a technician to the patient's specifications.

   Eyeglass prescriptions always have a spherical power, calculated by a technician to the patient's specifications.

9. The woman is on a diet. She hopes to reduce her body fat by 5%. She walks for exercise each day.

   Dieting and walking, she hopes to reduce her body fat by 5%.

10. Youths drink too much soda and sugared beverages. They are missing essential nutrients and the benefits of water.

    Youths drink too much soda and sugared beverages, missing essential nutrients and the benefits of water.

EXERCISE 6-14 Revise these sentences to ensure more specific expression and to ensure a positive "can-do" tone. These are sample sentences only. Yours will vary.

1. For this procedure, there are eight steps that must be carried out.

   This procedure has eight steps.

2. It is assumed that this individual is a hypochondriac.

   This individual is a hypochondriac.

3. There is a dental assistant who tells everybody how important brushing and flossing are to do.

   Dental assistants stress the importance of brushing and flossing.

4. He wants to try the task even if it is difficult.

   He will attempt the difficult task.

5. My coworkers are lazy when the boss isn't around.

   My coworkers lack motivation when the boss is not present.

6. Some patients are so picky.

   Some patients are very particular.

7. That sputum stinks.

   That sputum is malodorous.

8. He has to pee a lot.

   He urinates frequently.

9. I hate to lift heavy items.

   I dislike lifting heavy items. *or* Lifting heavy items is a challenge for me.

10. That is not my job.

    That task is outside my scope of duties.

UNIT PROOFREADING EXERCISES

Read the following passage and make corrections for errors in punctuation, spelling, syntax, exact language, and other sentence errors.

Mononucleosis is referred to as "mono" or the "kissing disease." ~~And~~ (It) is a viral infection~~. It~~ (that) is common in older teenagers and young adults~~. I believe it is most commonly~~ characterized by a sore ~~sore~~ throat and fatigue. Other ~~sympotoms~~ (symptoms) include weakness (,) dizziness(,) swollen lymph ~~glans~~ (glands)(,) and an in ~~larged~~ (enlarged) spleen. It is diagnosed by a blood test. This disease may last several weeks ~~or so~~. There is no specific ~~treat ment~~ (treatment) ~~accept~~ (except) rest (,) plenty of fluids(,) and ~~aspiring~~ (pain relievers) for body aches. If infected, ~~glasses and silverware should not be shared~~. (a person should not share glasses and silverware).

UNIT REVISION EXERCISES

Revise these sentences to improve their content and style.

1. The man, who is a dermatologist, encourages his patients to drink at least 64 ounces of water each day.

   The dermatologist encourages his patients to drink at least 64 ounces of water each day.

2. There is not a single reason for his unexplainable illness.

   No single reason explains his illness.

3. The man wanted to capture each moment with his grandchildren, so he videotaped them each time they visited him in the hospital.

   Wanting to capture each moment with his grandchildren, the man videotaped them each time they visited him in the hospital.

4. It is important that we exercise daily and avoid too many junk foods.

   Daily exercise and avoidance of junk food is important.

5. I believe that my struggle with trying to quit smoking has affected my lifestyle.

   My struggle with trying to quit smoking has affected my lifestyle.

UNIT 6 SELF-CHECK

Identify the phrase in each sentence. Underline and label each phrase. Use the following labels: appositive phrase *(AP)*, gerund phrase *(GP)*, infinitive phrase *(IP)*, participial phrase *(PaP)*, prepositional phrase *(PP)*, and verb phrase *(VP)*.

Patient Bob was admitted to the emergency room. Complaining of stomach pains,
(PP) *(PaP)*

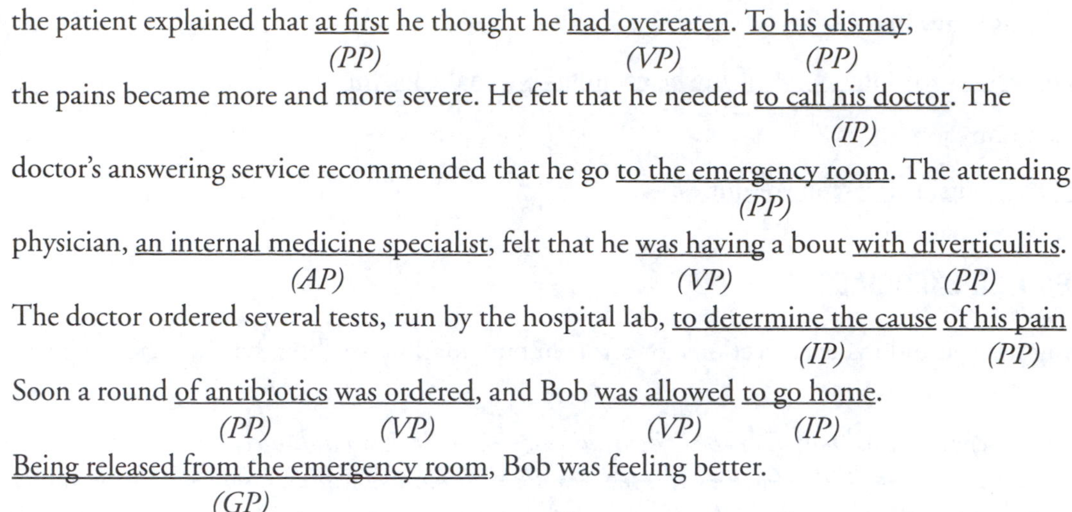

the patient explained that at first he thought he had overeaten. To his dismay,
(PP) *(VP)* *(PP)*
the pains became more and more severe. He felt that he needed to call his doctor. The
(IP)
doctor's answering service recommended that he go to the emergency room. The attending
(PP)
physician, an internal medicine specialist, felt that he was having a bout with diverticulitis.
(AP) *(VP)* *(PP)*
The doctor ordered several tests, run by the hospital lab, to determine the cause of his pain
(IP) *(PP)*
Soon a round of antibiotics was ordered, and Bob was allowed to go home.
(PP) *(VP)* *(VP)* *(IP)*
Being released from the emergency room, Bob was feeling better.
(GP)

UNIT 7: PARAGRAPH BASICS

EXERCISE 7-1 Label the parts of the paragraph below. Use the following labels: topic sentence, support sentence, and concluding sentence.

The development of ultrasonography has played a major role in noninvasive test procedures for diagnostic purposes. Ultrasonography is a technique that reflects high-frequency sound waves off internal tissues. A transducer, a detection device, locates and converts ultrasonic waves into electrical impulses. These impulses are then displayed on a video monitor and can be recorded for future evaluation. Ultrasonography is easy, inexpensive, and quick to administer. Little or no risk is presented to the patient. With this diagnostic technique, we are able to see internal tissue images, although not always clearly, without having to conduct time-consuming and expensive exploratory surgery. Patients and healthcare professionals alike benefit from this innovation.

Topic sentence: *The development of ultrasonography has played a major role in noninvasive test procedures for diagnostic purposes.*

Support sentences: *Ultrasonography is a technique that reflects high-frequency sound waves off internal tissues. A transducer, a detection device, locates and converts ultrasonic waves into electrical impulses. These impulses are then displayed on a video monitor and can be recorded for future evaluation. Ultrasonography is easy, inexpensive, and quick to administer. Little or no risk is presented to the patient. With this diagnostic technique, we are able to see internal tissue images, although not always clearly, without having to conduct time-consuming and expensive exploratory surgery.*

Concluding sentence: *Patients and healthcare professionals alike benefit from this innovation.*

EXERCISE 7-2 Review these topic sentences. Mark whether each is effective or ineffective.

1. Healthcare is an important subject. ☐ effective ☒ ineffective
2. Without a solid patient–client relationship, the healthcare provider may be limited in understanding the patient's needs. ☒ effective ☐ ineffective
3. I really want to be a medical assistant. ☐ effective ☒ ineffective
4. More research into the links among diet, exercise, and genetics will provide answers to a means of slowing the onset of chronic heart disease. ☒ effective ☐ ineffective

5. I think that the healthcare industry is booming. ☐ effective ☒ ineffective
6. Most people do not know that secondhand smoke kills 38,000 American each year.
   ☒ effective ☐ ineffective
7. Drug-addicted babies have a right to a safe home environment and excellent medical care.
   ☒ effective ☐ ineffective
8. Communicable diseases aren't common today. ☐ effective ☒ ineffective
9. A trip to the magazine aisle helped me realize that healthcare offers vast career choices.
   ☐ effective ☒ ineffective
10. Germs are bad. ☐ effective ☒ ineffective

EXERCISE 7-3 Write a topic sentence of your own for each topic below. Use the guidelines to assist your writing. Answers will vary; see your instructor for guidance.

EXERCISE 7-4 Develop one of the above topic sentences into a paragraph. Answers will vary; see your instructor for guidance.

EXERCISE 7-5 Write a test-question response in paragraph form. Choose <u>one</u> and respond. Answers will vary; see your instructor for guidance.

UNIT PROOFREADING EXERCISES

Read the following paragraph. Correct any errors in the grammar, punctuation, and paragraph format.

Pinworms are tiny(,) threadlike worms. They infect the digestive tract of young children. (Pinworms are common) ~~Common~~ among 4- to 6-year-old children, but anyone can become infected. Pinworms live in the upper portion of the intestine(,) and they travel outside the anus to lay their eggs~~. Which~~ (, which) occurs at night and causes the child to itch. These eggs are able to live outside the body for days on clothing and bedding(,) and this is how other family members can become infected. If a child scratches the rectum area and then sucks his thumb~~[;]~~ (,) reinfection occurs. If a parent suspects an infection, he or she should enter the bedroom at night and shine a flashlight on the ~~child~~ (child's) anus. The light will make the worms move back to the anus. ~~Over the counter~~ (Over-the-counter) remedies exist. Wash bedding and sleeping clothes. Encourage hand washing and keep fingernails short. In a severe case, the child may complain about stomach pains and experience a ~~lost~~ (loss) of appetite.

UNIT REVISION EXERCISES

This paragraph is in response to a test question on a first-quarter exam. You may edit and revise the paragraph in any way that improves it to meet the guidelines for effective paragraph writing. Write the revision on lined paper.

Assignment: Select one medical diagnostic technique and discuss its application in healthcare. This paragraph need not be overly technical, since it is not a research assignment.

Ultrasound

This is a fairly recent technology. With this invention, certain tests are affordable and practical for both the patient and the practitioner. Ultrasound has different velocities these differ in density and elasticity with different tissues. Ultrasound is a technique that has changed medicine. Ultrasound transmits sound waves through body tissues and records the echoes as the sounds encounter other objects within the body. The use of ultrasound is noninvasive. Ultrasound can be used to measure the size and shape of some internal organs. It is commonly used for monitoring fetuses. Ultrasound can detect abnormalities. Ultrasound is painless. Ultrasound does not harm the internal organs or a fetus. Ultrasound is also used in physical therapy. It has been know to help circulation and regeneration of tissue. Ultrasound requires specialized equipment but it can be used in a variety of ways.

One revision possibility is:

Ultrasound

Ultrasound is a recently developed technology. With this invention, certain tests are affordable and practical for both the patient and the practitioner. Ultrasound has different velocities; these differ in density and elasticity with different tissues. Ultrasound is a technique that has changed medicine. Ultrasound transmits sound waves through body tissues and records the echoes as the sounds encounter other objects within the body. The use of ultrasound is noninvasive. Ultrasound can be used to measure the size and shape of some internal organs. It is commonly used for monitoring fetuses. Ultrasound can detect abnormalities. Ultrasound is painless and does not harm the internal organs or a fetus. Ultrasound is also used in physical therapy. It has been known to help circulation and regeneration of tissue. Ultrasound requires specialized equipment, but it can be used in a variety of ways.

UNIT 7 SELF-CHECK

1. Draw a sketch of a well-developed paragraph. Label the three important parts and any distinguishing features that a paragraph should have.

Topic sentence ______________________________
Support sentences ______________________________
____
______________ Concluding sentence ______________

2. Imagine you are in a test situation. Relying on the information you have today and your personal experiences in healthcare, select one of the topics below and write a paragraph. Ensure varied sentence structure and adequate support.

   a. Answers will vary; see your instructor for guidance.
   b. Answers will vary; see your instructor for guidance.

3. Answers will vary; see instructor for guidance.

UNIT 8: WRITING SKILLS WITH DEFINITION

EXERCISE 8-1 Complete the chart for the medical terms below. You might need a medical dictionary. These terms will be used later in this unit.

Term	Class/Group	Distinguishing Features
polyp	tumor	a growth with a footlike appendage that attaches itself to organs such as the nose, rectum, or uterus
gastroscopy	examination	an inspection of the inside of the stomach using a gastroscope
scabies	infestation	condition caused by a skin mite that creates itching and a rash and is spread by skin contact
fulguration	procedure	a means to destroy tissue by using a long, high-frequency electrical spark
dyspnea	a condition	difficulty breathing or labored breathing
epistaxis	a condition	a nosebleed that occurs spontaneously or as a result of an infection
arrhythmia	a state or condition	an irregular beat or lack of rhythm, as in an irregular heartbeat
stridor	sound	a high-pitched, harsh sound during inspiration, indicating an upper airway obstruction
splenography	a procedure	a radiographic image of the spleen
dysphagia	a condition	difficult swallowing or an inability to swallow

EXERCISE 8-2 Draft sentences for the above terms that use word clues as a means of signaling definition. These are sample answers; your answers will vary.

1. polyp *A polyp is a tumorlike growth that is characterized by a footlike attachment; these growths occur in the nose, rectum, colon, and uterus.*
2. gastroscopy *A gastroscopy is a medical procedure that uses a gastroscope to view the interior of the stomach.*
3. scabies *Scabies is a contagious parasitic infection caused by the itch mite and it is characterized by itch and a rash.*

4. fulguration *Fulguration is a medical procedure that uses a long, high-frequency electrical spark to destroy tissue.*

5. dyspnea *Dyspnea is the condition of having difficult or labored breathing caused by physical exertion or a medical condition.*

6. epistaxis *Epistaxis is the medical term for a nosebleed, which may be spontaneous or as a result of an infection.*

7. arrhythmia *Arrhythmia is the condition of having an irregular or a lack of regular beat, as with the heart.*

8. stridor *Stridor is a high-pitched, harsh sound during inspiration, indicating an upper airway obstruction.*

9. splenography *Splenography is a medical procedure of taking a radiographic image of the spleen.*

10. dysphagia *Dysphagia is the medical condition of not being able to swallow or difficulty in swallowing water and/or food.*

EXERCISE 8-3 Read the sentences below. Determine each sentence's purpose in the paragraph and label as follows: topic sentence *(TS)*, supporting sentence *(SS)*, or concluding sentence *(CS)*.

1. *CS* *In summary, the cardiac cycle is the sequence that keeps blood moving from the veins, through the heart, into the arteries, and through the body.*
2. *TS* *Studies have shown that lactase deficiency may be congenital, resulting from prematurity, or it may be acquired.*
3. *CS* *Thus, lactose intolerance may be controlled by modifying the diet or taking medication.*
4. *TS* *The cardiac cycle is the sequence of events that occur in one heartbeat.*
5. *SS* *Next, the atria, upper heart chambers receiving venous blood, relax and the ventricles, lower heart chambers pumping blood to the body, contract.*
6. *TS* *Pneumonia is a bacterial infection of the lungs.*
7. *SS* *Lactose intolerance is the inability to digest lactose resulting from the deficiency of the enzyme lactase.*
8. *TS* *Many bacteria can cause pneumonia; streptococcus pneumoniae is the most common cause.*

EXERCISE 8-4 Write a definition paragraph. Choose one of the following terms or concepts and define it in a paragraph. You will need to rely on the Internet or other reference materials to locate information.

a.–f. Answers will vary; see your instructor for guidance.

UNIT PROOFREADING EXERCISES

Proofread the following paragraph. Locate and change any errors in grammar, usage, sentence structure, and punctuation.

Quitting smoking is one of the most important things you can do for ~~you~~ (your) health. There ~~is~~ (are) a lot of methods to help smoker(s) quit. One method is the nicotine patch. ~~They are~~ (This method uses) patches that release nicotine into the bloodstream in through the skin. The patch helps some smokers gradually withdraw from the nicotine ~~addict.~~ (addiction.) It is one method that helps smokers who have the withdrawal symptoms of headaches (,) anxiety(,) depression (,) and insomnia. By combining the patch and a smoking cessation program(,) a smoker (has an increased chance) ~~chances~~ for success (.) ~~can be increased.~~

UNIT REVISION EXERCISES

The paragraph below has many problems. Some sentences are awkward; others are out of order. Some sentences are run on, while others may be fragments. Revise this definition paragraph so that it is a good example of a definition paragraph. Use the checklist presented in this unit to ensure an effective paragraph.

The test for TB includes a skin test. Also saliva sample and a chest X-ray. It is called TB. Others inhale the bacteria. Sometimes it takes up to two years for a person to develop active TB. When people with TB cough or sneeze the infected bacteria become airborne. Tuberculosis is a contagious disease. It is caused by bacteria that infects the lungs. Others never do. Active TB is known for having the symptoms of weight lost, fatigue, fever, persistent cough, and general malaise. They create small areas of inflammation. Drug treatment for active treatment of TB is available it may take 6 to 12 months to cure. If not treated a person can die from TB. It can spread to other body parts. Especially to the brain, kidneys, and bones. The bacteria multiply.

One possible revision:

The test for tuberculosis, also called TB, includes a skin test, saliva sample, and a chest X-ray. Tuberculosis is a contagious disease. It is caused by bacteria that infect the lungs. The bacteria multiply. They create small areas of inflammation. It can spread to other body parts, especially to the brain, kidneys, and bones. When people with TB cough or sneeze(,) the infected bacteria become airborne. Others inhale the bacteria. Sometimes it takes up to two years for a person to develop active TB; others never do. Active TB is known for having the symptoms of weight loss, fatigue, fever, persistent cough, and general malaise. Drug treatment for active TB is available (, but) the disease may take 6 to 12 months to cure. If not treated (,) a person can die from TB.

UNIT 8 SELF-CHECK

1. What are the three parts of a formal definition sentence or paragraph?

a. term

b. class

c. distinguishing features

2. You may use a medical dictionary. Write a sentence definition for: [Sample answers; yours will vary.]

   a. comedo

   A comedo is a skin lesion characterized by a closed white papule called a whitehead, or an open form called a blackhead, often found on the face, chest, or back.

   b. pediculosis

   Pediculosis is the medical condition of having the parasitic infection of head lice or body lice that lay eggs in the hair or on the body and live off dead skin cells.

3. Choose one of the terms below. Draft a definition paragraph of your own. You may use any reference books you choose to gather your notes. This paragraph needs to be your own definition of the term. Use the definition checklist to assist you in editing the paragraph.

   a.–e. Answers will vary; see your instructor for guidance.

UNIT 9: WRITING SKILLS WITH SUMMARIES

EXERCISE 9-1 Read the passages below and then write a summary sentence for each, capturing the main idea of the passage.

Diabetics often have problems with their feet. One reason is that the peripheral nerves are damaged by poor circulation. The legs and feet are often affected because these are farthest from the heart's action; thus, blood circulation may be limited. Furthermore, abnormal blood glucose levels can damage blood vessels and nerves that take nourishment and nerve signals to the legs and feet. This damage then leads to the limbs becoming numb, feeling less pain, and having difficulty healing. With the loss of sensation, an individual may be unaware of foot sores or injuries. The feet then become ulcerated and infected. So, limb and foot care are important to maintain proper circulation and foot health.

Summary sentence: Answers will vary; see your instructor for guidance. One possible answer is: *Diabetics often have problems with their feet because of peripheral nerve damage and the loss of feeling in their legs and feet.*

Pain is an alarm system that gets our attention. Pain can signal that something has gone wrong with our bodies. It is a basic symptom of inflammation and can help an individual figure out what is wrong with his or her body. Pain comes in various sensations: throbbing, stabbing, or aching. Pain may be localized or generalized. Pain can be acute or chronic in nature. Furthermore, it can be mild or severe. Pain works as a help signal to pay attention to our bodies.

Summary sentence: Answers will vary; see your instructor for guidance. One possible answer is: *Pain, in its varying degrees, is a symptom that allows an individual to know that something is wrong with his or her body.*

Nosebleeds (epistaxis) are common occurrences. When the tiny capillaries inside the nose rupture, a nosebleed occurs. A nosebleed can be caused by simply blowing one's nose, having a cold or an allergy, being in cold or extremely hot and dry weather, or being hit in the face or nose. Usually pain does not accompany a nosebleed. Nosebleeds may have a small trickle of blood or produce severe and sudden bleeding. Nosebleeds are usually handled by first aid at home. So, although a nosebleed can be unsettling, usually it is nothing severe and can be managed by home care.

Summary sentence: Answers will vary; see your instructor for guidance. One possible answer is: *Nosebleeds, or epistaxis, result from a spontaneous event or an infection that makes the tiny capillaries inside the nose bleed; usually nosebleeds are handled with home care.*

EXERCISE 9-2 Choose one of the assignments below to complete.

1.–2. Answers will vary; see your instructor for guidance.

EXERCISE 9-3 Consider the skills that you have gained from work and college. Then develop a table of transferable skills. Answers will vary; see your instructor for guidance.

People Skills	Patient Care	Leadership	Recordkeeping

EXERCISE 9-4 Using the words in the table above, draft a sample resumé highlighting your specific skills to a job opening in your field. Use the commercially available resumé software to format your prose. Draft a resumé in any of these styles that markets your skills. Answers will vary; see your instructor for guidance.

EXERCISE 9-5 Draft a cover letter that applies for a position and that includes key elements of your resumé and transferable skills list. Answers will vary; see your instructor for guidance.

EXERCISE 9-6 Draft a sample thank-you note that is a follow-up to the cover letter and interview process. Answers will vary; see your instructor for guidance.

UNIT PROOFREADING EXERCISES

Proofread the following letter and make the needed changes in grammar, spelling, and punctuation.

This letter of application is for the post of Licensed practical nurse that was advertised in The Chronicle on Sunday November 7 2004. The listing noted that the position required a respondsive and responsible individual to provide home health care needs to a retirement community. Having worked first as a home health care aide, I begin my health career by supporting my patients in the privacy of there own homes. I am licensed and trained in several areas that support issues such as end-of-life care, family counseling grieving and handling the wide variety of insurance paperwork. My luv for the elderly is what attracts me to the post.

One possible answer:

This letter of application is for the post of licensed practical nurse that was advertised in *The Chronicle* on Sunday, November 7, 2004. The listing noted that the position required a responsive and responsible individual to provide home healthcare needs to a retirement community.

Having worked first as a home healthcare aide, I began my health career by supporting my patients in the privacy of their own homes. I am licensed and trained in several areas that support issues such as end-of-life care, family counseling, grieving, and handling a wide variety of insurance paperwork. My love for the elderly is what attracts me to this post.

UNIT REVISION EXERCISES

Read the following application to be a volunteer at a local hospital. Make any corrections necessary to ensure a professional and accurate application. Neatly add corrections to the application.

Meadowview Hospital Volunteer Application		
Name	Gretchen smith	
Address	23414 12th street West	
City, State, Zip	Los Angeles, CA 27654	
Home Phone	(213) 555-0100	
Work Phone		
Cell Phone	(753) 555-0199	
E-mail Address	smartgirl@yahoo.com	
Availability	☐ Weekday Mornings ☐ Weekday Afternoons ☐ Weekday Evenings Other Specific Times ______	☐ Weekday Mornings ☐ Weekday Afternoons ☐ Weekday Evenings
Available Start Date	Imediately	

Interested Area for Volunteering	☒ Clerical Tasks ☐ Customer Service ☐ Decorating Committee ☐ Family Support ☐ Fundraising ☐ Gift Shop	☐ Magazine Sorting ☐ Mail Delivery ☐ Phone Bank ☐ Reception Area ☐ Special Events ☐ Visitation Committee
	Other nope	
Special Skills and Qualifications		
Summarize special skills, qualifications, and attributes that you have gained through employment or previous volunteer work		
I am really fast typist and I like to do office work. Like filing, printing, mailing, and answerwering fones. I have recently retired. I need to so something.		
Summarize your previous volunteer experience		
I wanna get started giving back to the community. I have done charity work through my previous job and that inspires me to do more. I participate in "Senior walk-a-thong" for Alzhomiers research and "The Relay for Life" cancer benefit for the passed five years. I am active in my church.		
I affirm that the information in this application is true and complete.		
Signature /Date	GS	

Was the previous volunteer application to volunteer complete and helpful to the person reviewing the application? Answers vary; ask your instructor for guidance.

Note: The application was incomplete and had many spelling errors. Time available was not provided nor was availability. It was not dated. Rewrite the application below so that it is correct.

Meadowview Hospital Volunteer Application	
Name	Gretchen smith
Address	23414 12th street West
City, State, Zip	Los Angeles, CA 27654
Home Phone	(213) 555-0100
Work Phone	n/a
Cell Phone	(753) 555-0199
E-mail Address	smartgirl@yahoo.com
Availability	☒ Weekday Mornings ☐ Weekday Mornings ☒ Weekday Afternoons ☐ Weekday Afternoons ☒ Weekday Evenings ☐ Weekday Evenings Other Specific Times

<table>
<tr><td>Available Start Date</td><td colspan="2">Immediately</td></tr>
<tr><td>Interested Area for Volunteering</td><td>☒ Clerical Tasks
☒ Customer Service
☒ Decorating Committee
☒ Family Support
☒ Fundraising
☒ Gift Shop</td><td>☐ Magazine Sorting
☐ Mail Delivery
☐ Phone Bank
☐ Reception Area
☒ Special Events
☐ Visitation Committee</td></tr>
<tr><td></td><td colspan="2">Other ____________________</td></tr>
<tr><td colspan="3">Special Skills and Qualifications</td></tr>
<tr><td colspan="3">Summarize special skills, qualifications, and attributes that you have gained through employment or previous volunteer work</td></tr>
<tr><td colspan="3">I type 75 WPM and I like to do office work such as filing, printing, mailing, and answering phones. I have recently retired. I want to continue to work in the areas that I have strong skills.</td></tr>
<tr><td colspan="3">Summarize your previous volunteer experience</td></tr>
<tr><td colspan="3">I want to get started giving back to the community. I have done charity work through my previous job and that inspires me to do more. I participated in "Senior walk-a-thon" for Alzheimer's research and "The Relay for Life" cancer benefit for the past five years. I am active in my church. Working as a volunteer is something that I enjoy because of my sense of social justice.</td></tr>
<tr><td colspan="3">I affirm that the information in this application is true and complete.</td></tr>
<tr><td>Signature /Date</td><td colspan="2">Gretchen Smith December 12, 2005</td></tr>
</table>

UNIT 9 SELF-CHECK

1. What two important skills are used when writing summary sentences or paragraphs?
   a. restating the main idea
   b. paraphasing

Revise each of the following job-related statements so that each appears professional and effective for applying for a job. Add content and improved language.

2. I wanna to be a certified nursing aid because my friends said it was a good job.

   I am interested in being a certified nurse's assistant because of my desire to help the elderly and those who are vulnerable; furthermore, I have strong care-giving skills.

3. Thanks so much for considering my application.

   Please consider my application for the position of registered nurse for your trauma center; I look forward to hearing from you soon.

4. I am really interested in this position.

   This post as a dental assistant is what I have trained for, and I am ready for the busy work environment that your practice offers.

5. This is the reason that I think this job is perfect for me.

   As a massage therapist, I will help the company promote its philosophy of customer well-being and work as a team member to increase business.

6. Can you please call me for an interview?

   I may be reached at 203-555-0100 for an interview or further questions about my applications.

Read the job application summary of Mr. Fred Peterson and revise the summary to clarify any ideas that would assist him in presenting himself to the prospective employer:

> How can you tell us about yourself that might not be clear from your job application?
>
> First of all, I do like all people. I wanna travel all over the world and meet people. I spoke Spanish. I participate in local health care charities. I got into the health care field as a nurses aid becus my aunt was old and needed a lot of care so I sort of started to help her out. Then I took a course and learned the skills I needed to work in a long-term care facility.

7. What are the apparent weaknesses presented in this summary?
   - The language is not formal. Oral grammar is used.
   - Spelling errors
   - Weak content

One possible revision:

> How can you tell us about yourself that might not be clear from your job application?
>
> People are my passion. I enjoy traveling and meeting new people. I speak Spanish. I participate in local healthcare charities. My entry into the healthcare field was as a nurse's assistant. Initially I provided home healthcare for my aunt who needed care; Then I took a course and learned the skills I needed to work in a long-term care facility. My future goal is to become a registered nurse.

8. Write a summary paragraph form this table of information. The information is in no particular order.

What are head lice?	What else should I do?	How are head lice spread?
Lice are tiny insects that are gray, brown, or black. Lice crawl through hair. Lice lay eggs called nits on the hair shaft close to the scalp. Nits hatch in about 6 days. Nits are oval and attached to the hair shaft. They are easier than lice to spot.	*Check all members of the household. Treat all family members who have lice. Notify your child's school or daycare. Wash all combs, brushes, and hair clips in soapy water (above 129°F) for at least 10 minutes. Launder by washing and heat drying* *(continued)*	*Anyone can become infested by head-to-head contact, by wearing another person's hat or using his or her comb or brush or bedding or by sharing clothing.*

	all clothing and bedding used by the infested person in the 48 hours before treatment for lice. Vacuum furniture and carpets and change the vacuum bag thereafter.	
How can lice outbreaks be prevented?	**How do I treat hair to get rid of lice?**	**What are symptoms of head lice?**
Check you child's hair weekly for lice or nits. Do not share combs, brushes, or clothing; store items separately at school; wash clothing and bedding.	*Lice and their eggs can be treated with Nix; follow package instructions exactly.*	*Itching of the scalp is the most common symptom.*
What if lice come back?	**Where can I get more information?**	**What is the medical name for head lice?**
You may reapply Nix again after 7–10 days; this is not usually necessary.	*Call your family doctor or public health department.*	*Pediculosis*

Nix is a registered trademark of the Warner-Wellcome Company.

Answers will vary; see your instructor for guidance.

UNIT 10: WRITING SKILLS WITH PROCESS/SEQUENCE

Exercise 10-1 Your texts have procedures, certain patient care routines, or equipment setup or sterilization techniques in them. Select one of these and read it several times. Then write down the steps in sequence. Not only will this help you learn the individual steps, but it will also help you memorize the order of the steps. Answers will vary; see your instructor for guidance.

Exercise 10-2 Draft an *instructional* process paragraph on one of the following processes. Answers will vary; see your instructor for guidance.

Exercise 10-3 Draft an *informative* process paragraph on one of the following processes. Answers will vary; see your instructor for guidance.

Exercise 10-4 Think about a task that you will do or are learning how to do to be a healthcare professional. Illustrate it in a task-flow diagram. Answers will vary; see your instructor for guidance.

UNIT PROOFREADING EXERCISES

Compare the task-flow diagram with the paragraph below it. Assume that the task-flow diagram is the accurate information. Circle the inconsistencies in the paragraph. Then rewrite the paragraph so that it accurately describes the task-flow diagram.

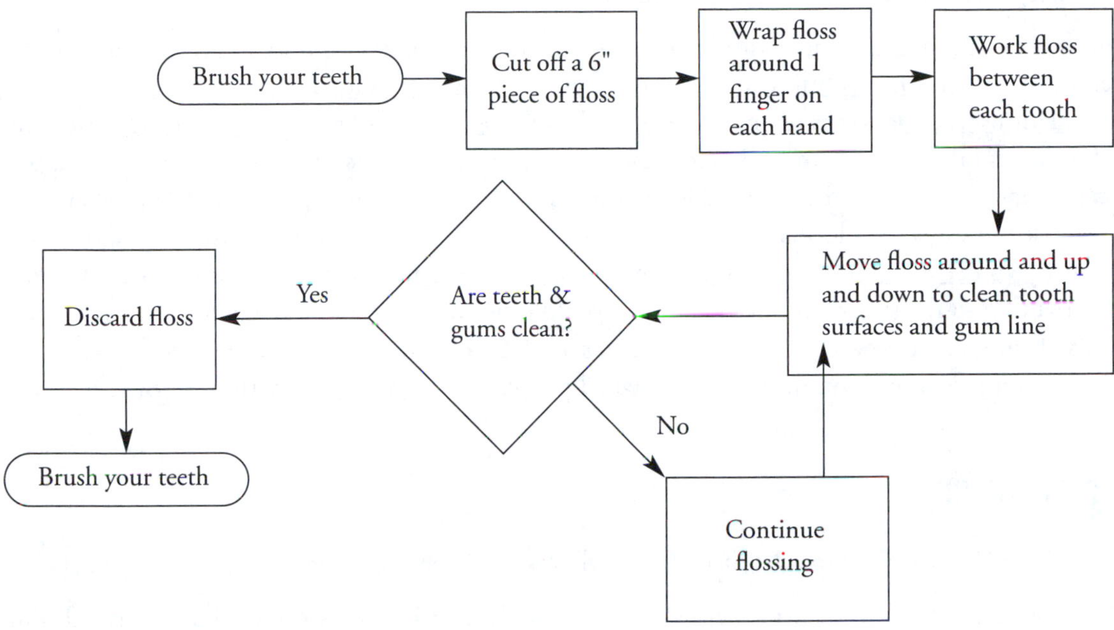

Step-by-Step Flossing

> *First brush your teeth. Wrap a piece of floss between two fingers. The floss should be cut into a six-inch piece. Push floss down, around, and back and forth between the teeth. Continue flossing. If the gum is cleaned, brush teeth. Discard floss.*

One possible revision:

First, brush your teeth. Then cut off a six-inch piece of floss. Wrap the floss around one finger on each hand. Work the floss between each tooth. Move floss around and up and down to clean tooth surfaces and gum line. Check to see if the teeth are clean. If they are, discard floss. If the teeth are not cleaned, continue flossing until they are.

UNIT REVISION EXERCISES

Read the following paragraph and make the following changes. First, reorder sentences that may be out of order. Then, add transition words to add clarity between the steps.

> Stress must be managed. One definition of stress is a human being's response to physical, intellectual, or emotional pressures. If stress is endured for long periods of time, the human body uses its defenses, and it will enter a stage of exhaustion or extreme fatigue. Stress has three fundamental stages: alarm, resistance, and exhaustion. Another definition is the mind's and body's reaction to either imagined or real threats, events, or situations. A situation is defined as stressful by our perception of the stimulus creating the stress.

The body's first reaction to stress is a physical reaction called fight-or-flight. There is a sudden release of the hormones epinephrine and norepinephrine. This hormone release increases the blood flow to the muscles, which, in turn, improves muscle strength and mental ability. Another state is called resistance. The body begins to cope by adapting to the stress, and this appears to build resistance to the stress. In other words, your body handles the stress better. Stress is an internal reaction to the events that all people encounter; what matters is how we respond to it.

Stress must be managed. One definition of stress is a human being's response to physical, intellectual, or emotional pressures. Another definition is the mind's and body's reaction to either imagined or real threats, events, or situations. A situation is defined as stressful by our perception of the stimulus creating the stress. Stress has three fundamental stages: alarm, resistance, and exhaustion. The body's first reaction to stress is a physical reaction called fight-or-flight. There is a sudden release of the hormones epinephrine and norepinephrine. This hormone release increases the blood flow to the muscles, which, in turn, improves muscle strength and mental ability. In other words, your body handles the stress better. The second state is called resistance. The body begins to cope by adapting to the stress, and this appears to build resistance to the stress. Finally, if stress is endured for long periods of time, the human body uses its defenses, and it will enter a stage of exhaustion or extreme fatigue. Thus, stress is an internal reaction to the events that all people encounter; what matters is how we respond to it.

UNIT 10 SELF-CHECK

1. Read the following sentences; then arrange them in sequential order.

5 **a.** Place the thermometer in the healthcare facility's chemical solution for the prescribed time or in 90% alcohol.

4 **b.** Dry the thermometer after rinsing it with water.

1 **c.** Clean the thermometer with soap or detergent solution, rubbing it with firm strokes.

6 **d.** Use a soft, clean tissue or gauze to wipe the thermometer.

3 **e.** Rinse the thermometer under cold running water.

7 **f.** Rinse the thermometer in warm water after disinfecting it and store in a dry place.

2 **g.** Hold the tissue or gauze at the thermometer's stem and wipe downward toward the bulb. Twist firmly as you wipe downward.

2. Select a process you will do as a healthcare professional. It can be something such as changing a colostomy bag or calculating a medication dosage. List the steps in sequential order from start to finish. Then draft a paragraph from this process. Answers will vary; see your instructor for guidance.

UNIT 11: WRITING SKILLS WITH ANALYSIS

Incident of April 2, 2007

I was just workin and I noticed Bob staring at me. Then he whispered something to Fred. I got mad becuz they always be talking and goofin off when de boss is in a meeting and I am doing all the work. It's notfair so I yelled at those dudes, but latter I told em I was sorry.

EXERCISE 11-1 List the facts and opinions in the incident report of April 2, 2007 above.

Incident Report: April 2, 2007	
Facts	**Opinions**
I was working	They are always goofing off
Bob whispered something to Fred	I am doing all the work
I yelled at them	It is not fair
I told them I was sorry	
Bob was staring at me	

Incident of April 2, 2007

On Monday April 2, 2007, at 9:30 a.m., I was making patient beds in Wing C on the second floor. I was distracted by the whispering of Bob Maestro and Fred Johnson who appeared to be making fun of me. I knew that Mr. Brown was in a meeting, and I could not leave my work area to locate the Head Nurse. I raised my voice at them to try to let them know that I did not appreciate their behavior. That was a poor choice of actions on my part. I immediately apologized to Fred and the patients and staff in the hallway.

EXERCISE 11-2 List the facts and opinions in the incident report of April 2, 2007, above.

Incident Report: April 2, 2007	
Facts	**Opinions**
Monday April 2, 2007, at 9:30 a.m., I was making patient beds in Wing C on the second floor	Bob Maestro and Fred Johnson appeared to be making fun of me.
Mr. Brown was in a meeting.	That was a poor choice of actions on my part.
I could not leave my work area to locate the Head Nurse.	
I raised my voice at them to try to let them know that I did not appreciate their behavior.	
I immediately apologized to Fred and the patients and staff in the hallway.	

EXERCISE 11-3 Revise the following memos, notes, and incident reports. You may add any details to clarify and improve the communication.

Answers will vary; see your instructor for guidance.

Original Note	Revision
Fix this stupid copier—ASAP!	12/03/05 Ms. Brown, This morning I noticed that the copier was not working. I tried to dislodge a jammed item, but I still could not get the copier working. Please contact the service representative to repair the machine. Thanks so much, Ted

Original Note	Revision
3/4/06 John— Last night my dad nearly keeled over. He's in a bad way. I need to take some time off. Jerry	3/4/06 John, Last night my father was very ill. I was in the emergency room with him all night. He has been admitted for observation. I will not be able to come to work today, and I will call about tomorrow. Jerry

Original Note	Revision
12/12/07 We don't have enough volunteers for the cookie drive and blood pressure check clinic this Saturday outside Safeway. Come on guys and do something!	12/12/07 We are asking for volunteers to help us in our cookie drive and blood pressure check clinic this Saturday outside Safeway. Your teamwork is outstanding, and it makes us unique in this community. Please contact Thelma in Human Resources to sign up for a shift. Thank you, Junior

Original Note	Revision
Incident Report I entered Room 110 and before I new it I was on the floor. I was sittin in a puddle of water. How it got there I don't have a clue. I can't believe our maintenance people are so lazy anyway. Susan	Incident Report for 11/05/06 fall: I entered Room 110, and I slipped and fell on the floor. A puddle of water had collected on the floor. I have a sprained ankle, and I will probably have a bruise or two. Although I am not badly hurt, we need to ensure that this type of accident is avoided. Please remind the janitorial service to ensure that all floors are dry. Susan Keene, RN

EXERCISE 11-4 Read the situation below and then complete the incident form adding information to complete each line. For example, you will need to provide a name and address on this incident form. Answers will vary; see your instructor for guidance.

On Saturday afternoon at 12:25, I was delivering a hot food tray to Mrs. Brown in room 234. As I turned into room 234, a visitor, Frieda Berkshure, was exiting the room. I did not see Ms. Berkshure coming out of the room, and I ran into her, spilling the tray and upsetting Mrs. Brown. The dishes dropped off the tray, and hot water sprayed everywhere. No hot water hit Frieda Berkshure or Mrs. Brown. As I picked up the broken glass, I cut my hand across the palm. I immediately applied pressure. I called a nurse to assist me. I went to the doctor immediately and had fifteen stitches put in my right hand. I returned to work and told Mr. Smith what happened. He told me to take the rest of the day off.

CITY HOSPITAL INCIDENT REPORT

Name of individual(s) involved: *Your name*

Place of incident: *City Hospital Room 234*

Date and time of incident: *Saturday, January 7, 2006 at 12:25 p.m.*

Incident was reported to: *The head nurse, Mrs. Louise Johnsten*

Description of the incident:
I was delivering a hot food tray to Mrs. Brown in room 234. As I turned into room 234, a visitor, Frieda Berkshure, was exiting the room. I did not see Ms. Berkshure coming out of the room, and I ran into her, spilling the tray and upsetting Mrs. Brown. The dishes dropped off the tray, and hot water sprayed everywhere. No hot water hit Frieda Berkshure or Mrs. Brown. As I picked up the broken glass, I cut my hand across the palm. I immediately applied pressure.

Follow-up action needed:
I went to the doctor immediately and had fifteen stitches put in my right hand. I returned to work and told Mr. Smith what happened. He told me to take the rest of the day off. I need to fill out an absence report.

Report submitted by: *Your name* Date of report: *date*

EXERCISE 11-5 Read the situation below and then complete the incident form, adding information to complete each line. For example, you will need to provide a name and address on this incident form. Answers will vary; see your instructor for guidance.

I was driving the company vehicle to pick up some office supplies from Office Central. When I returned to the lot, I did not see that the garbage dumpster had been moved. I hit the edge of the dumpster with the right fender of the vehicle. I dented the fender. There is a 9-inch dent in the fender of the car. I was not hurt. The dumpster did not get damaged. The fender has the dent plus some paint was scraped off in the process. My insurance company is Allstate and my policy number is TR-45783-234. I was on duty when this accident occurred. I reported this accident to my supervisor, Bob Gregory, and to the head of maintenance, who handled the Pacific Rim Care and Reh. Center's vehicle. I had no witnesses.

PACIFIC RIM CARE AND REHABILITATION CENTER ACCIDENT AND INCIDENT REPORT

Please print in black ink

Personal Information	
Full Name of Injured Person *Your name*	
☒ Employee ☐ Visitor ☐ Trainee ☐ Public ☐ Contractor ☐ Other	
Address: *12354 48th Avenue South*	
Portland, Oregon 97895	
Job Title: *Activities Director*	Date of Birth: *May 11, 1954*
Work Phone: *204-555-0100*	Home Phone: *204-555-0199*

Accidental/Incident Details		
☒ Accidental Injury ☐ Threatening Behavior/Verbal ☐ Physical Violence ☐ Other (Specify): ____________		
Date: *5/23/05*	Time: *12:15 pm*	Documentation ☐ yes ☒ no
Witnesses: *None*		
What was the injured person doing at the time of accident? *I have no injuries.*		
If employee, how long in this position? *12 years*		
Who was in charge? *Nurse Bernie Cousins*		
Were others involved? ☐yes ☒no If yes, specify:		
Was equipment involved? ☒ yes ☐ no If yes, specify: *When I returned to the lot, I did not see that the garbage dumpster had been moved. I hit the edge of the dumpster with the right fender of the vehicle. I dented the fender. There is a 9-inch dent in the fender of the car. I was not hurt. The dumpster did not get damaged. The fender has the dent plus some paint was scraped off in the process.*		
Were there injuries ☐ yes ☒ no If yes, specify:		
Were the injuries treated by a medical professional? ☐ yes ☒ no If yes, specify treatment:		
For employees:		
If absence from work expected, specify in days: *none*		
This information is correct and true as stated:		
Signature: *Your name*		Date: *May 23, 2005*

EXERCISE 11-6 Choose words from the chart below to complete the paragraph.

condition	yellow	symptoms	icterus
enters	bile	yellowing	jaundice

One of the *symptoms* of liver disease or problems is the *yellowing* of the skin. *Jaundice* is the name of the condition when the skin turns *yellow*. This *condition* is also known as *icterus*. A *bile* duct may be blocked. In this case, the bile *enters* the bloodstream.

EXERCISE 11-7 Use the words in the chart below to complete the fill-in-the-blank statements. The word should be consistent with medical use of the term and fit the context.

efficiently	procedure
in the room	immediately
warm	in turmoil
scraped	diet
will exhaust	dental

1. The procedure (*noun*) was performed by the technician.
2. The dental (*adjective*) procedure made the patient feel nervous.
3. The dental assistant scraped (*action verb*) the tartar from the bicuspid.
4. Meeting the family in the room (*prepositional phrase*), the head nurse ensured they were apprised of the patient's progress.
5. The surgical technologist returned to the surgery suite immediately (*adverb*).
6. The energy needed to breathe will exhaust (*verb phrase*) an ill person.
7. In turmoil (*prepositional phrase*), the staff cannot function efficiently.
8. The procedure was completed efficiently (*adverb*).
9. By watching your diet (*noun*), you will lose weight.
10. Warm (*adjective*) baths may help the patient feel more comfortable.

EXERCISE 11-8 Draft an analytical paragraph on *one* of the following topics. Answers will vary; see your instructor for guidance.

UNIT PROOFREADING EXERCISES

Read the following paragraph. There are five errors in word use. Locate them and make the corrections.

Leishmania is a ~~parasite~~ (parasitic) disease of the skin, viscera, or mucous ~~membrous~~ (membranes). Leishmaniasis is caused by leishmania, which is transmitted to people via the bite of infected female sand flies. Leishmania organisms infect and ~~reproduction~~ (reproduce) in the macrophages. These organisms are controlled by a T-cell mediated response. Leishmania cutaneous is a chronic ~~ulerationing~~ (ulcerating) nodular skin lesion prevalent in tropical regions. Treatment options are somewhat limited and available only ~~throught~~ (through) the Centers for Disease Control by a doctor.

UNIT REVISION EXERCISES

Revise the sentences to ensure the correct use of the terms. You may find using a medical dictionary to be helpful. Each sentence has one error that is underlined. Write the correction on the line provided.

1. Integumentarial is derived from the Latin term for covering. Integumentary
2. He is scheduled for an endoscopy examination. endoscopic
3. Under a microscope, kidney tissue revealed approximately 1 million nephrons filtering units. nephritic
4. Necrotis is the death of cells, tissues, or organs. Necrosis
5. Assessing the posttrauma stress patients requires a lot of documentation. posttraumatic stress
6. A phlebography or venography is a radiographic of the veins to identify and locate abnormalities in the veins of the lower extremities. radiography
7. Impetigo is an inflame skin disease that is marked by pustules that become crusty and rupture. inflammatory
8. Selecting a prime care physician from all the available family medicine doctors is a challenge. primary care physician
9. Pavor nocturnus is a condition of anxious of the young or aged; it occurs during the night and is known as "night terrors." anxiety
10. Excising prostate tumors is one of the new cryosurgical that Dr. Wills has perfected. cryosurgeries

UNIT 11 SELF-CHECK

1. Use the words below to fill in the blanks:

air	wheezing	asthma	reach
increase	constriction	illness	airways
SOB	hospitalization	severe	inflammatory

Asthma is an inflammatory respiratory illness, which is characterized by mild to severe difficulty in breathing. Constriction and swelling of the airways and an increase in mucous secretion close the smaller passages. When this occurs, air cannot reach the lungs. Wheezing occurs as the air is forced through the narrowed passage. An asthma attack can create shortness of breath (SOB) and may lead to hospitalization.

2. Fill in the parts of speech. Put an *X* in a box if a form of the term does not exist.

Noun	Verb	Adjective
medicine	medicate	medicated
allergy	*X*	allergic

excision	excise	excised
diagnosis	diagnose	diagnostic
idiopathy	*X*	idiopathic

3. Write an analytical paragraph. Use a health-related topic from your personal life or one social issue that interests you. Keep an objective point of view. Answers will vary; see your instructor for guidance.

UNIT 12: WRITING AN ESSAY

EXERCISE 12-1 Look at the topic and essay question below. Underline the background information. Then, underline the question twice. Box any key words that could be used in an effective thesis statement in response to this assignment.

Healthcare offers individuals a wide variety of career options and ladders for professional growth. Many people decide on the healthcare field because they like to help others. Others have experienced good quality of care in the field and want to contribute to the profession. How did you decide upon the specific field you chose in healthcare? Write a composition in which you detail your choice, how you made the decision, and why. Be specific and use examples to support your views.

EXERCISE 12-2 Read the following essay topics. Draft a thesis statement for these topics. Answers will vary; see your instructor for guidance.

EXERCISE 12-3 Choose one of the thesis statements that you developed from the previous pages. Draft an introductory paragraph. Remember that the thesis statement should be the final sentence in the introductory paragraph. Indent the first line. Answers will vary; see your instructor for guidance.

EXERCISE 12-4 Continue with the topic you chose in Exercise 12-3. Draft two support paragraphs for this topic. Answers will vary; see your instructor for guidance.

EXERCISE 12-5 Write a concluding paragraph that continues your essay from 12-3 and 12-4. Answers will vary; see your instructor for guidance.

EXERCISE 12-6 Choose *one* of the following topics and draft an essay. Answers will vary; see your instructor for guidance.

Exercise 12-7 Using a professional journal, locate one article of interest. After reading the article, write an annotated bibliography. Answers will vary; see your instructor for guidance.

Exercise 12-8 Use the following information to make an APA-formatted reference citation.

1. Frederick Fell Publishers, Inc. By Marianne Pilgrim Calabrese. Hollywood, California. 2004. So you want to be a Nurse? pp 23–26.

   Calabrese, M. P. (2004). *So you want to be a nurse?* Hollywood, CA: Frederick Fell Publishers, Inc.

2. JADA–Journal of the American Dental Association November 2004. pp. 1537–1542. The integration of clinical research into dental therapies : the role of the astute clinician. Volume 135. Sharon M. Gordon DDS, MPH, PhD Raymond A. Dionne DDS, PhD.

   Gordon, S. M., & Dionne, R. A. (2004, November). The integration of clinical research into dental therapies: The role of the astute clinician. *Journal of the American Dental Association, 135,* 1537–1542.

3. Asthma Treatment Guidelines and Medications pp 32–37 April. Pharmacy Times April. Lauren S. Schlesselman. (2000, April)

   Schlesselman, L. S. (2000, April). Asthma treatment guidelines and medications. *Pharmacy Times,* 32–37.

4. Janice M. Boutotte, RN, CS, MS. Volume 29 Number 3, 1999 March. pp 34–39. Nursing 99 Keeping TB in check.

   Boutotte, J. M. (1999, March). Keeping TB in check. *Nursing 99, 29,* 34–39.

5. 2000. Salvatore Tocci, New York. Franklin Watts. Down Syndrome.

   Tocci, S. (2000). *Down syndrome.* New York: Franklin Watts.

Exercise 12-9 Use the following information to make an MLA-formatted reference citation.

1. Frederick Fell Publishers, Inc. By Marianne Pilgrim Calabrese. Hollywood, California. 2004. So you want to be a Nurse? pp 23–26.

   Calabrese, Marianne Pilgrim. So You Want to Be a Nurse? Hollywood, CA: Frederick Fell Publishers, Inc., 2004. 23–26.

2. JADA–Journal of the American Dental Association November 2004. pp. 1537–1542. The integration of clinical research into dental therapies: The role of the astute clinician. Volume 135. Sharon M. Gordon DDS, MPH, PhD Raymond A. Dionne DDS, PhD.

   Gordon, Sharon M., and Raymond A. Dionne. "The Integration of Clinical Research into Dental Therapies: The Role of the Astute Clinician." Journal of the American Dental Association 135 (2004): 1537–1542.

3. Asthma Treatment Guidelines and Medications. pp 32–37. April. Pharmacy Times 2000. Lauren S. Schlesselman. April 2000.

   Schlesselman, Lauren S. "Asthma Treatment Guidelines and Medications." Pharmacy Times Apr. 2000: 32–37.

4. Janice M. Boutotte, RN, CS, MS. Volume 29 Number 3, 1999 March. pp 34–39. Nursing 99. Keeping TB in check.

   Bouttotte, Janice M. "Keeping TB in Check." Nursing 99 29.3 (1999): 34–39.

5. 2000. Salvatore Tocci, New York. Franklin Watts. Down Syndrome.

   Tocci, Salvatore. Down Syndrome. New York: Franklin Watts, 2000.

UNIT PROOFREADING EXERCISES

Read the following annotated bibliography and make changes in punctuation, spelling, and format. Cross the errors out neatly and replace with the corrections.

S. Trossman. (February 2004,). Want a safer patient care. *American journal of Nursing*, 104(2)
In this article the author states improving working conditions of nurses produce quality patient care. This is organized and well written article.

In the February 2004 issue of *American Journal of Nursing* an article entitled, "Want Safe Patient Care"? Susan Trossman notes that the (IOM) Institute of Medicine puts emphasize on the improving working conditions of nurses to provide a better patient care. Both IOM and (AN) American Nursing Association acknowledge that proper patient care is in danger when there is understaffing makes it difficult for the nurse to provide quality bed side care when working long hours. Therefore the IOM points out recommendations that could solve these problems.

The IOM advices that hospitals and long term facilities inforce a staffing level for every shift and unit that meet the needs of each patient such as scheduled procedure, emergency care, or discharging practices. Cross-trained staff members can be valuable assets for this flexibility. The nursing staff should play an active role in designing and implementing a staffing system that will ensure patient safety. The IOM also addresses overtime by recommending state governments to ban 12-hour shifts. In addition IMO encourages nursing schools and health organization to teach the danger of fatigue caused by prolonged working hours on patient safety.

The article has value to nursing because it shows the great danger of inadequate patient care caused by unsatisfactory working conditions of nurses. Plus, the nurse must be an advocate for the patient whenever the patient's needs are not meet because of understaffing. In conclusion this articles is importance because it deals with the solutions to solve poor working conditions of nurse to provide quality patient care.

Adapted from Azeb Zeleke, LPN Student

Answers will vary. This is one possibility:

Trossman, S. (2004, February). Want a safer patient care? *American Journal of Nursing*, 104(2).

In this article, Trossman states that improving working conditions of nurses will produce quality patient care. This is an organized and well-written article.

In the February, 2004, issue of *American Journal of Nursing*, in an article entitled "Want Safe Patient Care?" Susan Trossman notes that the Institute of Medicine (IOM) emphasizes improving the working conditions of nurses to provide the best patient care. Both IOM and American Nursing Association (ANA) acknowledge that proper patient care is in danger if there is understaffing because this shortage in personnel makes it difficult for the nurse to provide quality bedside care when working long hours. Therefore, the IOM points out recommendations that could solve these problems.

The IOM advises that hospitals and long-term facilities enforce a staffing level for every shift and unit that meets the needs of each patient, such as scheduled procedures, emergency care, or discharging practices. Cross-trained staff members can be valuable assets for this flexibility. The nursing staff should play an active role in designing and implementing a staffing system that will ensure patient safety. The IOM also addresses overtime by recommending that state governments ban 12-hour shifts. In addition, IMO encourages nursing schools and health organization to teach the danger of fatigue on patient safety caused by prolonged working hours.

The article has value to nursing because it shows the great danger of inadequate patient care caused by unsatisfactory working conditions of nurses. Plus, the nurse must be an advocate for the patient whenever the patient's needs are not met because of understaffing. In conclusion, this article is important because it deals with the solutions to poor working conditions of nurses to provide quality patient care.

UNIT REVISION EXERCISES

Revise the following annotated bibliography. Neatly rearrange the information or make the corrections.

Trossman, S. (2004, February). Want a safer patient care? *American Journal of Nursing*, 104(2).

In this article, the author states improving working conditions of nurses produces quality patient care. The article is organized and well-written.

In the February 2004 issue of *American Journal of Nursing*, in an article entitled "Want Safe Patient Care?" Tossman notes that the Institute of Medicine (IOM) puts emphasis on improving working conditions of nurses to provide the best patient care. Both IOM and American Nursing Association (ANA) acknowledge that proper patient care is in danger when understaffing makes it difficult for the nurse to provide quality bedside care when working long hours. Therefore, the IOM makes recommendations that could solve these problems.

The IOM advises that hospitals and long-term facilities enforce a staffing level for every shift and unit that meets the needs of each patient, such as scheduled procedures, emergency care, or discharging practices. Cross-trained staff members can be valuable assets for this flexibility. The nursing staff should play an active role in designing and implementing a staffing system that will ensure patient safety. The IOM also addresses overtime by recommending state governments ban 12-hour shifts. In addition,

IOM encourages nursing schools and health organization to teach the danger of fatigue to patient safety caused by prolonged working hours.

The article has value to nurses because it shows the great danger of inadequate patient care caused by unsatisfactory working conditions. Plus, the nurse must be an advocate for the patient wherever the patient's needs are not met because of understaffing. In conclusion, this article is important because it deals with the solutions to poor working conditions of nurses and ways to provide quality patient care.

UNIT 12 SELF-CHECK

Write a three-page research paper on a current healthcare issue, a specific drug, a medical organization, or a public policy. Use APA formatting and type the paper. Provide at least five reference citations. Ask a peer to edit it for you. Make revisions. Submit it to the instructor for scoring. Use the following Self-Check list for research papers in your proofreading and revision.

Answers will vary.

Index

Note: Answers for exercises appear in boldface